本教材为安徽省教育厅2022年度新时代育人质量工程项目(研究生教育)结题成果之一，项目编号为2022ghjc043

安徽省研究生教育质量工程项目
安徽省省级研究生规划教材
医学英语新医科课程群系列教材

医学英语写作

Medical English Writing

U0250633

主　编　刘维静　袁　远
副主编　刘娅敏　孙　娟　葛　雪
编　者：（按姓名首字母排序）
　　　　葛　雪　李洪伟　刘维静
　　　　刘娅敏　庞　炜　孙　娟
　　　　汪　媛　徐　燕　薛　艳
　　　　袁　远

南京大学出版社

图书在版编目(CIP)数据

医学英语写作 / 刘维静，袁远主编. -- 2 版. -- 南京：南京大学出版社，2024.4
ISBN 978 - 7 - 305 - 27507 - 4

Ⅰ. ①医… Ⅱ. ①刘… ②袁… Ⅲ. ①医学－英语－写作 Ⅳ. ①R

中国国家版本馆 CIP 数据核字(2024)第 000458 号

出版发行　南京大学出版社
社　　址　南京市汉口路 22 号　　　　　邮　编　210093
书　　名　医学英语写作
　　　　　YIXUE YINGYU XIEZUO
主　　编　刘维静　袁　远
责任编辑　裴维维　　　　　　　　　编辑热线　025 - 83592123

√参考答案
√课件申请

照　　排　南京南琳图文制作有限公司
印　　刷　常州市武进第三印刷有限公司
开　　本　787 mm×1092 mm　1/16　印张 15.5　字数 430 千
版　　次　2024 年 4 月第 2 版　2024 年 4 月第 1 次印刷
ISBN 978 - 7 - 305 - 27507 - 4
定　　价　47.00 元

网址：http://www.njupco.com
官方微博：http://weibo.com/njupco
官方微信号：njupress
销售咨询热线：(025) 83594756

* 版权所有，侵权必究
* 凡购买南大版图书，如有印装质量问题，请与所购
  图书销售部门联系调换

前　言

　　《医学英语写作》自2013年出版以来,结合医学生英语学术写作实际需求,以普通医学院校专业英语教学实践为基础,一直作为医学院校硕士研究生和临床本硕一体化"5+3"学生的基础英语写作教材。现根据这十多年教材使用经验和诸多兄弟院校师生及同行反馈,对教材进行修订。修订后的教材主要呈现以下特色:

1. 注重英语写作"微技能"训练

　　英语写作"微技能",是指从词汇特征和句型结构入手,辅助学习者掌握学术英语语言特色,从前期选词造句基本功开始,到后期段落、篇章整体构建。此次修订版仍保留了原版教材注重"微技能"训练的特色,在第一部分"医学英语写作微技能"中详细讲解学术词汇选用与构词特征、名词化现象、平行结构等常见写作句式,为篇章学术论文写作打下扎实基本功。

2. 更新、替换大部分例句和例文

　　医学技术发展日新月异,教材中所用例句也应紧随时代发展。现借此修订机会,根据平时备课和教学实践经验,将原教材中大部分例句和例文进行替换,尽量从一些国际知名期刊选取材料,以确保例文的权威性。

3. 精心设计丰富多样的练习

修订版教材除了进行大量例句和例文分析之外,还紧扣讲解内容设计了形式更为多样的练习,如改错、判断、排序、英汉互译、找关键词等,使学习者真正得到写作技能的训练,逐步培养学术写作思维,提升学术写作能力。

4. 讲解应用文写作,满足实际工作和学习考试需求

随着医学科学技术的进步发展,医学生对外交流的机会和需求大大增加,参加医学英语水平考试(METS)的人数也逐年上升,此次修订版增加了医学英语应用文写作讲解和练习,包括个人简历、申请信函、会议通知、学术报告等内容,以满足更多医学生学术写作的实际需求。

写作非一日之功,需要不断地练习和总结,才能有所进步。希望本次修订版教材能为广大医学院校师生和其他医务工作者系统、熟练掌握医学英语学术写作基本技能、拓展学术写作思维提供帮助。

由于编者水平有限,本教材不足之处难以避免,敬请广大师生和学习者在使用过程中对发现的问题进行批评指正。

编　者

2024 年 3 月

目　录

第一部分　医学英语写作微技能

第二部分　医学英语写作语篇技能

第三部分　医学英语应用文写作

第一部分

医学英语写作微技能

第一章　学术词汇基本特征概述

因医学英语具有说明性（informative）、解释性（explanatory）、思辨性（analytical）和展望性（speculative）等特征，医学英文学术写作不仅需遵循英语书面语的一般规则，在词汇的选择和运用方面还需要将医学专业词汇与一般性学术写作词汇相结合，从而把理论基础、临床观察，乃至现状—问题—实验/观察—结果—讨论的研究过程转化为规范化的语言和图表。英语非母语的作者需要了解英语学术写作的基本词汇特征、与汉语学术写作词汇选择之间的差异，从而用英语合理措辞，产出合乎范式的学术文献。

第一节　学术写作中的术语应用

英语医学学术文本给人最直观的印象之一是术语繁多，术语的领域专业度高。近年来，快速发展的生物医学科技和信息技术手段与医学研究的结合使文献涵盖的信息量呈指数级增长，新术语层出不穷，跨学科借词日渐增多。

1.1　术语与非术语普通词的并用

非母语作者在选词方面往往矫枉过正——过分强调使用术语、大词等所谓书面用语——在实际操作中，合乎专业习惯和语域要求的普通词其实并不少用。当然，部分俗词未形成惯用，且与术语相比，其构词能力和屈折变化相对有限，因此在构句时的功能稍逊一筹。

对非母语作者来说，术语词汇结构复杂、音节多，与非术语词汇的差别显而易见，比较容易区分；应该留意的是非术语单词——普通词汇、方言和俚语等口头语，其中普通词汇一般可以用于学术文体，而其他口头语则不宜用于学术写作。某些词典或翻译软件缺乏标注，没有描述词汇的语域特征，写作者可能仅从语义考虑，导致选词失当，将方言俚语用于学术写作，应予注意。下表展示了若干组例词：

	Terminologies(术语)	Plain words(普通词)	Colloquialism(口头语)
气管	trachea	air way	windpipe
高血压	hypertension	high blood pressure(HBP)	pressure
流感	influenza	flu	grip/gripe/grippe
细菌	bacterium	/	germ
呕吐	emesis	vomiting	throwing up/puking
瘀伤	contusion	bruise	chafe
切口	incision	cut	gash
梗阻	obstruction	blockage	jam

普通词汇用于医学语境,进而成为普遍接受的术语,这样的例子并不少见。例如,普通词 murmur 原指"持续低而模糊的声音",用在 heart murmurs 中表示"心脏杂音";冠状动脉旁路移植术(coronary artery bypass grafting)中的普通词 bypass 原指工程建设领域为解决拥堵路段而修建的旁路,现在作为医学术语用来描述心脏手术,形象贴切,中文表述为"搭桥术"。再如,"牙关紧闭"可使用源于拉丁文的 trismus 表达,也可使用 lockjaw,只不过通过 PubMed 检索可知,近十年来后者使用的频率明显较低。

1.2 医学术语的规范化

1.2.1 医学术语的一词多式

拉丁/希腊/古法语等多样的词素来源、词素转写不统一、英式/美式拼写的差异等诸多因素使医学术语往往出现一词多式,或者拼写形式不统一。规范的术语不仅要拼写正确,更需要作者参考自己所在学科的论文写作规范,选用合适的单词或变体。

某些一词多式的术语在意义上几无差异,可以通用,例如,surgery 与 operation 被看作同义词;"四肢瘫痪"对应 tetraplegia/quadriplegia,两词可互换使用;lymph node 或 lymph gland 都表示"淋巴结";"注射"既可以表达为 injection,也常表述为 infusion。

但有些情况下,术语的不同形式指向的意义有别,例如"肺炎"对应英语术语 pneumonia 和 pneumonitis。在临床工作中,两词具体所指有别:pneumonia 特指感染引起的炎症,如 bacterial pneumonia(细菌性肺炎)、viral pneumonia(病毒性肺炎)、fungal pneumonia(真菌感染引起的肺炎);pneumonitis 所指较宽泛,可以指感染性肺炎,但更多的时候专指非感染引发的肺部炎症,例如 interstitial pneumonitis(间质性肺炎)。请看以下例句:

例 1:Farmer's lung is a type of hypersensitivity pneumonitis, which is a noninfectious allergic lung disease that is caused by inhaling mold spores in the dust from moldy hay, straw, or grain.

上例中，farmer's lung(农夫肺)指一种非感染性的肺炎，病因在于吸入霉菌孢子引发过敏反应，需用 pneumonitis 指称这种变应性肺炎。

1.2.2 医学术语的拼写变体

医学术语也存在英语/美语变体，英式拼写更注意保持这些源于古典语言词素的完整性，而美式英语的术语拼写倾向于删繁就简，不发音的字母有时被省略，使拼写更易于发音。例如，"呕血"haematemesis(英)/hematemesis(美)、"血红蛋白"haemoglobin(英)/hemoglobin(美)、"贫血"anaemia(英)/anemia(美)。从这三组词中可以看出，英式拼写完整地保留了转写自拉丁语的"血液"haemat-/haemo-，而美式英语为了发音的便利，将 ae 简写为了 e。同理，"麻醉"的美式拼写为 anesthesia，英式为 anaesthesia。

英式拼写中的 oe 对应美式拼写的 e，例如，"水肿"oedema(英)/edema(美)、"淋病"gonorrhoea(英)/gonorrhea(美)、"腹腔的"coeliac(英)/celiac(美)等等不一而足。

少数词尾也存在英语与美语的对应，英式的-our、-re、-logue、-ise 分别对应美式的-or、-er、-log、-ize。举例如下：

- 肿瘤：tumour(英)/tumor(美)
- 纤维：fibre(英)/fiber(美)
- 门类：catalogue(英)/catalog(美)
- 麻痹：paralyse(英)/paralyze(美)

1.3 医学术语的现时性

术语的嬗变伴随着医学的发展和观念的进步。有一部分医学术语逐渐陈旧，失去现时性，被作者们自然淘汰。历史上赫赫有名的结核病就几易其名，现代医学诞生以前，古希腊人称其为 phthisis，东方称之为"痨"，中世纪的西方称之为 scrofula，英法称其为 king's evil，因为当时人们普遍认为国王若肯触碰病人，患者就会痊愈。18 世纪始称 consumption 或 white plague，直至 19 世纪下半叶，微生物学先驱发现结核杆菌，该病才逐渐定名为 tuberculosis。及至今日，tuberculosis 及其缩写 TB 已成为规范表达。

新近出现的术语也在经受着审视，仍以肺炎为例，从构词角度来说，pulmonitis 也是可行的表达之一，然而通过 PubMed 检索可知，检索结果指向 pneumonia，且 pulmonitis 在 20 世纪 90 年代之后罕有采纳，已不具现时性。同样，近期文献通常使用 stroke 表达"卒中"，而少用 apoplexy；如需使用后者，一般需加定语，指出发病位置，例如 pituitary apoplexy，即"垂体卒中"。

一些带有强烈种族主义色彩或污名意味的术语如今也随着人文精神的深入而被废止，例如"先天愚型"的英文表达为 Down's syndrome。尽管"疯牛病"一词依然存在于大众媒体，mad cow disease 却不属于科学用语，科学文献一律使用 Creutzfeldt-Jakob disease。

这一进步尤其以精神医学领域最为突出，cretinism、amentia、insanity、black dog 等词曾广泛用于描述精神疾患，现今都已不再用于医学学术语境，取而代之的是所指明确、范畴清楚、态度中立的新术语：congenital hypothyroidism、intellectual disability、psychosis、depression。

与此同时，西方医疗消费化的加深使得某些术语的更替有偏离正道的风险，例如将"医护人员"称为 care providers 而非 doctors and nurses；"临床判断"（clinical judgement）改为 evidence-based practice。这类新术语是对消费社会模态的迎合，看似先进，实际矫枉过正，脱离了医学的本质，已经为业内有识之士所批评，不应模仿。

1.4 术语的缩写

术语缩写包括：① 单词截短，如：temp.、Prof.、approx.；② 计量单位，如 mL、h、s、min；③ 化学名称，如"钠"Na^+、"钠离子通道"Na^+ channel、"钠钾 ATP 酶"Na^+-K^+-ATPase；④ 首字母组合词，如 AIDS、ELISA、NATO、ANOVA，这些组合往往可读作单词，例如 Extracorporeal Membrane Oxygenation 的首字母组合词为 ECMO，当成一个单词读作/ekməʊ/；⑤ 首字母缩写，如 HPLC、WHO、ATP、DNA，这样产生的字符串不能当作单词来读，只能逐个读出字母音。医学论文写作最常见的是第四种缩写。

尽管原则上论文标题应避免使用缩略词，但计量单位、化学名称、标准缩写以及行业内广为人知的标准缩写可以直接用在论文的标题，以及摘要、正文中；而非标准的缩写第一次在文本中出现时都应该完整地写出来，再加括号，给出缩写形式，例如 the American Psychological Association（APA）。此外，句子最好不要以缩写开头，作者可以通过完整拼写术语或改换词序加以调整。

例 2：CABG was performed after aspirin was administered，and the use of clopidogrel during follow-up was allowed but not mandatory.

可修改为：Aspirin was administered before CABG，and the use of clopidogrel during follow-up was allowed but not mandatory.

【参考译文】冠脉搭桥前给予阿司匹林，后续治疗使用氯吡格雷，但不是强制使用。

拉丁文缩写属于约定俗成的缩写词，不需要给出定义但需注意区分大小写，如"医学博士"，拉丁文写作 Medicinae Doctor，缩写为 M. D.，使用大写形式；"每日"写作 Q. D.；etc.、i. e.、e. g. 和 cf. 则习惯小写。严格来说拉丁缩写仅用于插入和补充材料中（如表格、注释或列表），在一篇文章的正文里，应使用与之对应的完整英文单词，然而实际操作中破例甚多。

首字母缩写(initialism)尤其常见，它们可以减少字数，加速交流，便于拼写，易于记忆。然而医学文献的作者大量使用这一方法，创造出的缩略词就可能"撞脸"，导致歧义，例如，AMI 既可能指代治疗癌症的 amifostine（氨磷汀），也可指抗抑郁药 amitriptyline(阿米替林)；ED 可能指代疾病 eating disorder(进食障碍)，也可能指代外科手术 elbow disarticulation(腕关节断离术)。

为了适应期刊论文严格的字数限制,医学作者难免会使用缩略词或首字母缩写。少部分首字母缩略词和符号,如 DNA、PCR 和 cm,已经为读者熟识。然而,大多数非标准的、个人化的缩略词,其所指并不为读者熟悉,密集使用会极大地增加阅读难度,作者应当谨慎使用。

此外,作者自创首字母缩写时,还需避免与业已俗成的缩写雷同,导致歧义。例如 OCT 一般表示 over the counter,即"非处方药",一些眼科学者将 optical coherence tomography 也缩写为 OTC 则欠考虑;再例如 HM 常表示药物学的 herbal medicine,即"草药";"高度近视"英语表达为 high myopia,则无必要缩写为 HM。

1.5 跨学科借词

学科语言是学科发展和社会交流的产物,任何一种学科语言都或多或少受到关联学科的影响;术语的跨学科流动既是必然,也不少见。医学语言在规范化的过程中借入了相当数量的其他学科术语。

例词 1:remission
术语来源:*法学*
术语原义:*减轻或取消对刑事犯罪的处罚,即减刑或缓刑*
例句:The interest in this case is the recurrent intermittent retention of urine dependent upon remissions or exacerbations of anaemia in the course of a pernicious anaemia.

该例句是 PubMed 可检出的第一例对法学术语 remission 的应用,发表在 1907 年的《外科学年鉴》上,表示疾病的"缓解"。句中 remission 与 exacerbation 两词并置、词尾押韵,意思相反,remission 使用得恰如其分,描述了"一例恶性贫血患者贫血症缓解/恶化与其复发的间歇性尿潴留的相互关联"。该词在 20 世纪 70 年代后被医学作者广泛使用,出现了 spontaneous remission、complete remission、durable remission、clinical remission 等,具体实例如下:

a. A secondary outcome was remission of depression.

b. Focal segmental glomerulosclerosis in patients who are homozygous (or compound heterozygous) for two APOL1 variants is a rare, rapidly progressive disease with a very low likelihood of spontaneous remission of proteinuria.

c. The primary end points for induction (week 12) and maintenance (week 52) were clinical remission and endoscopic response.

医学在 20 世纪经历了爆发式发展,层出不穷的新术语被创造或从相关学科引入,来命名从机制原理到疾病诊疗的新发现。新千年以来,计算机技术与人工智能大举进入人类生活的各个领域。统计学、信息学、工程学领域的术语越来越多地出现在近年来的医学文献中。Algorithm(算法)、big data(大数据)、bioinformatics(生物信息学)等术语为医学研究者熟知。再如：

例词 2：ground truth

术语来源：机器学习

术语原意：地面现实，或基准现实，指比照真实世界的情况检查机器学习结果的准确性

例　句：The visual assessment also showed a good agreement between the automated segmented choroid and the manual ground truth.

在新语境中 ground truth 特指眼科学研究者"人工测量（脉络膜厚度）"，以比照机器自动测量的脉络膜厚度。

第二节　学术写作中的词汇替换

在不影响表意准确的前提下，合理进行词的替换，增加词汇多样性，这是英语书面表达的重要特征之一。医学学术论文，尤其是原创性论文和综述，词汇重复使用的频率原本就高，如不加注意，不提高词汇的多样性，语言贫乏的问题会格外突出。换词可降低阅读疲劳，增加文本的可读性。

学术写作进行词汇替换，提高词汇丰富程度的主要途径包括：单词的屈折与派生、近义词、普通词、代理词块（surrogate word chunks）、外壳名词（shell nouns）、上义词（hypernyms）替换。

2.1　单词屈折与派生

英语单词的屈折（inflection，又译作词形变化）指动词的时、体、态，名词、代词、形容词的性、数、格变化。经过屈折变化，单词的词性甚至意义都可能发生改变，在构造语句时也就具备了新的语法功能。

与此同时，单词通过添加前缀、后缀发生词形变化，则能产生与原有单词意义不同的新词，这种现象称为派生（derivation），是英语构词的重要途径。

单词的屈折形式与派生词一起构成词族，为写作提供了丰富的词汇资源。以单词 person 为例，其屈折和派生出的单词就包括：person's、persons、personal、personally、personalistic、personage、personalize、personalized、personalizing、personalization、personality、impersonate、impersonalization、depersonalize、interpersonal、intrapersonal、transpersonal 等等，不一而足。

汉语是典型的分析语，主要依靠词序、虚词等手段体现句中各成分的语法关系，较少依赖词本身的形态变化，因此汉语作者在使用英语组织语句时容易忽视词形变化，用词显得局促和机械。

例 1：Augmentation agents, or other antidepressants not included in the MGH

ATRQ, are qualified as a treatment failure if they failed to ameliorate <u>depression</u>, provided they had local regulatory approval as a treatment for major <u>depressive disorder</u>.

可以看出,如将画线词统一为 depression,则 antidepressant 可以换为 medications for depression,depressive disorder 可换为 depression,表意并无差别,但措辞单调。本句得益于屈折和派生词的使用,不仅表意清楚,词汇的丰富度也令人满意。

2.2 近义词替换

学术写作中非术语词汇的替换通常可借助近义词、代词、助动词等实现。用代词替换前文的名词或名词性词组,用助动词替换前文的动词或动词词组,需要注意指涉清楚,避免含糊,此处不再赘述;更重要的是,作者能够掌握丰富的近义词,灵活恰当地进行词的替换。下表列举的是四种词性的实词及其近义词,可以看出,例词与近义词意义基本吻合,替换十分方便。

例词	词性	意义	近义词
chance	名词	可能性	probability/likelihood/prospect
aggravate	动词	加重	worsen/intensify/exacerbate
urgent	形容词	急迫的	critical/crucial/exigent
rarely	副词	少见地	hardly/seldom

对于非母语作者来说,调动既往的词汇储备或借助近义词字典寻找近义词,选择与原词外延一致、内涵接近的词才可达成恰当的替换。但汉语作者对英汉词汇的内涵意义往往认识有限,导致近义词的选择失误。以形容词"瘦的"为例,与英文单词 thin 外延一致的近义词包括 underweight、slim、slender、skinny、lanky、scrawny、undernourished 等,但因内涵不同,用法也随之变化。

应该注意的是,underweight 作为技术性词汇,有明确的指标和参数,因此,最常为学者们使用,通过对《新英格兰医学杂志》(NEJM)已发文献的检索也证实了这一点,如:

例 2:Characteristics that were significantly associated with relapse were being <u>underweight</u> (defined as a weight that was ≥10% below the ideal body weight) at diagnosis, the presence of cavitation and bilateral disease on chest radiography, white race, and sputum-culture positivity after 8 weeks of treatment.

与此同时,slim 有时也被用来表示"清瘦的",但其内涵意义是 attractively thin,所以在 NEJM 检出的文献中,slim 多用来描述健康的或无明显病态的患者。

例 3:On examination, the patient was <u>slim</u> and appeared exhausted, without apparent physical distress.

形容词 slender 的内涵意义与 slim 相似,常指体量轻、身形苗条,同时也表示"截面周长与长度或高度相比偏小",因此,常用来描述细菌等微生物的形态。

例 4:Weight loss after a traumatic choking incident, which, in a patient with an already slender frame, resulted in a serious case of low body weight.

例 5:The organism's appearance was not suggestive of listeria, which typically appears small and slender on staining.

最为我们熟悉的单词 thin 往往暗含贬义,基本不用在医学论文里描述人的体格,而常用来描述"膈、膜、囊、纤维、血管、涂层"等厚度小、壁薄,或"黏液、溶液"稀薄。

例 6:Patients were instructed to apply a thin layer of cream once daily to cover psoriasis lesions completely.

单词 skinny 带有较强的贬义,不用于描述患者体格特征,而 scrawny 在 20 世纪 70 年代以后一般只用来描述动物。

单词 undernourished 在结构上与 underweight 相似,但强调营养的缺乏,因此要么用来描述饥饿或恶性疾病,要么用来描述营养不良的儿童患者。

例 7:A vicious cycle has been envisaged in which undernourished HIV-infected persons have micronutrient deficiencies, leading to further immunosuppression and oxidative stress and subsequent acceleration of HIV replication and CD4 + T-cell depletion.

2.3　术语的同义转换

术语因其单义性,从本质上排斥近义词的存在,实际上很难找到意义相同的另一个术语来替换,学术写作中往往依靠非术语普通词、代理词块、外壳名词、上义词/涵盖性术语等来改善行文单调的问题。非术语普通词已在本章第一节提及,现就后三种替换方法做简要介绍。

2.3.1　代理词块(surrogate word chunks)

如果难以找到一一对应的近义词进行替换,可考虑用若干单词构成的词块,对前文某个术语进行指代,这种词块起着代理原词的作用,被称为代理词块。

例 8:Many physicians recommend interrupting continuous anticoagulant therapy for dental surgery to prevent hemorrhage. In reviewing the available literature, there are no well-documented cases of serious bleeding problems from dental surgery in patients receiving therapeutic levels of continuous warfarin sodium therapy, but there were several documented cases of serious embolic complications in patients whose warfarin therapy was withdrawn for dental treatment.

在上述例子中,前句提及牙科手术前暂停抗凝药物,预防手术后的 hemorrhage,显然该术语特指较为严重的出血。Hemorrhage 作为术语,缺乏近义词,作者在后句中用词块 serious bleeding problems 进行指称。

再举一例,在一篇题名为"Long-Term Complications in Youth-Onset Type 2 Diabetes"的综述中,尽管"并发症"这一概念主要使用了术语 complication,如例 9 所示:

例 9:Among participants who had onset of type 2 diabetes in youth, the risk of complications, including microvascular complications, increased steadily over time and affected most participants by the time of young adulthood.

但作者仍采用了一些代理词块进行替换,来表达"并发症"之意:

例 10:Furthermore, serious cardiovascular events, although uncommon, occurred despite the young age of the participants.

例 11:Because the study offered no treatment or intervention in this phase, only adverse events related to study procedures were evaluated.

2.3.2 外壳名词(shell nouns)

外壳名词指一系列无具体所指的抽象名词,如 fact、theory、issue、idea 等,在特定语境中可用来指涉前文述及的具体内容,从而减少词汇或文本的重复。有学者按用途将外壳名词分为六类,见下表。

外壳名词的分类(Classification of shell nouns)		
分类(Classes)	例子(Examples)	
实际事实(Factual Fact)	issue　　point　　　　problem　　data　　　statistics　value level　　concentration　finding　　discovery　evidence	
语言学新闻(Linguistic News)	message　　report　　　question	
精神想法(Mental Idea)	theory　　notion　　belief　　　aim　　　　concept	
情态可能性(Modal Possibility)	truth　　　possibility　need　　　ability	
事件行为(Eventive Act)	move　　measure　　reaction　　implication　procedure	

例 12:Bans on gender-affirming care also refer to social contagion, a theory that has been used to describe the mode by which gender dysphoria "spreads" among the younger generation.

例 13:Decompressive craniectomy consists of removal of piece of bone of the skull in order to reduce intracranial pressure. The procedure has been shown to reduce mortality when used as a treatment for traumatic brain injury.

分别用 theory 和 procedure 指代两个例子中的医学术语 social contagion 和 decompressive craniectomy，避免了术语的重复使用。

2.3.3　上义词(hypernyms)

上义词是指在语义关系上处于上级的词汇，它的意思往往较为概括，向下延伸可包括一系列意义更加具体的词汇，这些具体的词汇称为下义词；有些时候，上下义关系可以等同于"纲要—实例"的关系。用上义词替代前文出现的下义词，是英语写作实现同义替换的重要方法之一。Malignancy 作为表"恶性肿瘤"的概括性术语，可以用来替换前文中的某种具体恶性肿瘤疾病，例如 sarcoma(骨肉瘤)、lymphoma(淋巴瘤)、central nervous system(CNS) tumor(中枢神经肿瘤)等。可以看出，这些疾病作为下义词时，可以被上义词 malignancy 替换，而当讨论深入微观层面时，这些疾病名称又可以与其具体分型构成上下义关系，并替换其下义词，因此上下义关系是相对的。

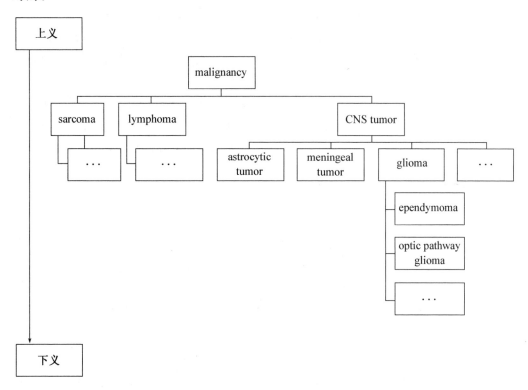

需要指出的是，使用上义词替换下义词并不一定逐级进行，跨级指代的例子屡见不鲜，例如用 hand condition(手部疾病)指代 symbrachydactyly(短指粘连畸形)，跨过了后者的直接上义词 rare congenital malformation(罕见的遗传性手部畸形)。

例 14：Furthermore, we defined a repertoire of lncRNAs possibly involved in <u>multiple myeloma</u>, as they meet the requirements of being both co-expressed and in close proximity to genes that have been described as relevant to this <u>neoplasia</u>.

例 15：C-reactive protein，SAP，and PTX3 bind various <u>bacteria，fungi，and viruses</u>，promoting innate immune responses to these <u>pathogens</u>.

第三节　学术写作中的几种重要词类

3.1　重视动词与介词

　　英语单词可分为实词和虚词两大类,毋庸置疑,任何文本主要依赖的都是传达信息的实词。非学术写作惯于大量使用修饰性实词——形容词、副词,对事物的状态、事件进行描述。但在学术写作时,尤其是在篇幅严格受限的期刊论文写作中,首先要确保研究事实和观点的完整表述,则要求倚重核心实词——名词与动词,减少单纯表达态度、情感、价值判断和责任等的修饰性语汇;同时,学术语篇的说服力主要来源于事实,论点需客观、语言需严谨,依靠修饰性语汇加强论述语气的做法只能适得其反,修饰性实词的使用不可避免地被进一步压缩。因此,写作时应特别留意不要过度修饰、前置修饰,减少冗余。

　　英语虚词不能单独充当句法成分,但有连接或附着各类实词的语法意义,其中一些词在汉语中无对应词,或用法大相径庭。汉语作者在进行英语构句时应特别注意对比英汉虚词的差异,其中容易受到母语负迁移干扰的两类词是介词和连词。

3.1.1　准确选择动词

　　不论英汉,句子意义中心是名词。但由于英语作为屈折语,语法信息需要通过动词的变形体现出来;相对而言,汉语形态标记欠发达,汉字不因时态或词性而变形,动词的正确形态是汉语作者需要面临的一个挑战。

　　下文的例 1 选自 *BMJ*（*British Medical Journal*）所载论文,文章比较了英美两份权威指南——美国的 Fleischner 指南和英国胸科协会（BTS）指南——在肺结节治疗领域的新观点。

　　例 1：In the case of multiple solid nodules，both the Fleischner and BTS guidelines <u>recommend</u> using the largest nodule to guide management. The Fleischner guidelines make specific recommendations for multiple nodules，and in particular <u>advocate</u> shorter intervals （3—6 months in the first instance） for medium-sized solid nodules，regardless of risk.

　　例句中的 recommend 和 advocate 虽然都表示"提议、建议",但所表语气的强弱有别,recommend 表示"因赞成而提出建议",在例子中表达了两大权威指南的一致意见,即仅利用患者肺部最大的结节指导治疗;另一个报道动词 advocate 强调的是"公开己方建议,通常是为了说服有异议的人",用这个词可以显示 Fleischner 指南对中型实体结节的单方面处理意见。经过分析可以看出,两个报道动词选词恰当,表意准确。

对汉语作者而言,用好动词极为重要,是正确表意的必备条件;选择恰当的动词可使表达干脆有力,避免再加副词进行修饰,保证语篇简洁准确。

从表述的内容来看,动词也可以分为具象动词和抽象动词两大类,当然学术写作的智性属性决定了抽象动词的广泛使用,但具象动词表意形象、表达有力,有助于把抽象概念诉诸相对易于接受的表达形式,受到母语作者的青睐,某些具体动词已经成为学界的标准表达或术语,被广泛使用。

例 2:Once triggered, a cascade of host responses <u>drives</u> sepsis, early critical care interventions to support organ system function and clear the causative pathogens are essential to patient survival.

谓语动词 drive 原义为"驱使、驾驶",显然比用抽象动词 cause 或 lead to 更加鲜明。

例 3:As regards patients <u>harboring</u> the mutations of BRAF, NRAS, KRAS, or DIS3 mutations, we identified the upregulation of 97 lncRNAs in DIS3 mutated samples.

该句中的 harbor 原指"像港口泊停船只一样给予某物庇护"(to provide a place, home, or habitat for),引申为"内含,含有"(to have within, contain)。如作者使用 have 一词,可以达到表意的目的,但语言表现力则有所削弱。

例 4:Unfortunately, artemisinin resistance has emerged in Southeast Asia, threatening these gains and potentially <u>derailing</u> current control efforts.

本句中,作者使用了 derail 一词,原义"脱轨",在此可引申为"干扰、破坏",用词十分生动。

总的来说,动词是英语句子的灵魂和语法的核心,合理选用动词可使表达更加直接、有力。

3.1.2 用对介词

从语言对比的角度来看,介词是汉英两种语言共有的词类,有些在意义和语法上具有可比性,但无论从句法功能和词汇意义的范畴来说,汉语介词都不如英语介词那么活跃,汉语介词的数量也远少于英语介词。注意使用介词,重视介词与实词的正确搭配是写出地道英语句子的一个前提。

以下是学术交流场合一些常用的介词与实词搭配:

搭配名词	in due course　solution to　on average　on the whole
搭配动词	account for　convince of　stem from　distinguish from
搭配形容词	related to　devoted to　aware of　dependant on

探讨医学问题时,表属性、范围、目的、条件的介词,或联结后置定语的介词,如 with、of、for、in 等用处很大。

例 5:A 7-year-old boy was brought to the emergency department <u>with</u> nausea, vomiting, and muscle weakness <u>for</u> the past several days.

例 6:The primary purpose <u>of</u> the final analysis was to perform formal statistical testing <u>of</u> overall survival.

此外,一般性书面体常用的并列句、复合句在医学期刊论文中也不鲜见,但存在字数限制的条件下,可以减词压缩,改为介词短语,增加医学文本的信息密度。

例 7:This is a retrospective cohort study of patients who were newly diagnosed with AML, and who received induction therapy at the First Affiliated Hospital of Anhui Medical University from April 2005 to October 2018.

观察例 7,发现 patients 有两个定语从句,第二个定语从句距离被修饰词较远,可以稍做修改。本句可改为:

This is a retrospective cohort study of newly diagnosed AML patients who received induction therapy at the First Affiliated Hospital of Anhui Medical University from April 2005 to October 2018.

例 8:The handwashing technique using soap in avian flu and also alcohol-based sanitizer is described.

受汉语限定词前置的影响,本句未能合理使用介词。全句仅使用了一个介词 in,且使用不当,无法与其后的名词成分搭配,句子显得别扭,需改为 in avian flu epidemic。通观整句,增加介词可以较好地调整词序,使表达自然。改为:

The technique of handwashing with soap or alcohol-based sanitiser in avian flu epidemic is described.

可以看到,正确使用介词不仅能够表意,更能将句子各个成分的逻辑关系凸显出来、合理连缀,写出符合英语句法要求的句子。

3.2　用词冗余问题

冗余分为积极冗余和消极冗余,前者又称合理冗余,指为了表达效果而正确得体添加的语言成分,属于修辞手段,而后者则是由于语言缺乏锤炼而导致的成分多余,又称为赘言,是需要修正的语病。本节探讨的是作为语病的冗余、成因,及修改思路。

学术写作过程中的词汇使用不当造成的局部冗余会削弱文本的流畅性,干扰写作意图的达成,更会显得作者表达能力有限、学术素养不高。针对汉语作者的母语习惯和新手作者的实际语言能力,写作一稿特别是修改稿件时可着重关注下列原因导致的冗余:形容词与副词、连接语、范畴词。

3.2.1　合理使用形容词/副词修饰语

英语形容词和副词在语法功能上与汉语相似,既不像英语句子里的名词要考虑数与格的问题,也不像动词要注意时与态的变化,是英语句子里形态稳定的成分,容易为汉语作者掌握并使用。然而,可能正是由于看似容易,形容词,特别是副词容易被汉语作者过量使用,导致行文累赘。从 unexpected surprise、overused cliche、universal panacea 来看,形容词的冗余主要表现为修饰语与名词意义的重叠;而在 very unique、completely eliminate、absolutely necessary 的表达中,形容词和副词的冗余源于过度修饰,或口语代入,这种语病经过推敲可以纠正。

例 9:The potentially superior antiplaque and better surface-active properties of amine fluoride and stannous fluoride containing mouth rinses were carefully investigated in a well-designed double-blind, crossover study in 10 healthy volunteers.

阅读例 9 可知,该句描述的是一项小规模的双盲实验,旨在测试某漱口水预防牙菌斑的效果和所含防蛀成分的活性。使用了 potentially superior、better 描述漱口水效果,使用 carefully、well-designed 强调实验的卓越,都属于不必要的修饰,有违科学写作客观扼要的宗旨。删去冗余的形容词和动词,该句可改为:A double-blind crossover study investigated the antiplaque and surface-active properties of amine fluoride and stannous fluoride containing mouth rinses in 10 healthy volunteers.

例 10:Amid pandemic-related disruptions in services, tuberculosis case notifications have decreased significantly and mortality has increased.

例 11:The prevalence of dementia is expected to rise significantly as the average life expectancy increases, but recent estimates suggest that the age-specific incidence of dementia is declining in high-income countries.

可以看出两个例子在描述增长/减少时使用了副词 significantly 以加强 decrease/rise 的表现力,这也是汉语作者惯常的做法,以上两例修改如下:

例 10 修改为:Amid pandemic-related disruptions in services, tuberculosis case notifications have plummeted and mortality has increased.

例 11 修改为:The prevalence of dementia is expected to soar as the average life expectancy increases, but recent estimates suggest that the age-specific incidence of dementia is declining in high-income countries.

3.2.2 连接语的误用

连接语(connectives)是让语句、段落与上下文相连接的功能性语汇,可以是连词、副词、介词、词组等,对于英文行文的逻辑建构十分重要,然而新手作者由于缺乏学术论文的写作思维和谋篇布局能力,在使用连接语时,易出现以下两个问题:一是追求语法对等,过度依赖与汉语对应程度高的连接语;二是用量呈极化发展:要么罕用,导致逻辑不清;要么过量使用,导致啰唆冗余。

先看追求语法对等造成的关联词滥用。汉语式的连接词习惯成对使用,例如"虽然……但是……""因为……所以……""一方面……另一方面……"等,如不加注意,很容易直译为 although ... but ... 、as ... so ... 、on the one hand ... on the other hand ... 等。

例 12:尽管无创呼吸支持技术是否是治疗急性呼吸衰竭的最佳选择仍存在争议,但无可否认的是经鼻高流量氧疗(high-flow nasal cannula, HFNC)已成为各种临床情况下行之有效且耐受性良好的呼吸支持技术。

例 13:由于干扰了正常的 OPN 调节作用,OPN 的阻断或沉默也可能会导致其他严重的不良反应,因此需要进一步研究,系统地比较这些治疗方法的局限性和可行性。

在人工智能和机器翻译蓬勃发展的今天,我们尝试将上述两个例子经由翻译软件转成英语,遂得到:

例 12 机器翻译:Although it is still debatable as to whether non-invasive respiratory support is the best option for acute respiratory failure, yet there is no denying that high-flow nasal cannula(HFNC)has emerged as a proven and well-tolerated respiratory support technique in a variety of clinical settings.

例 13 机器翻译:Because it interferes with normal OPN regulation, the blocking or silencing of OPN may also lead to other serious adverse effects, so further research is needed to systematically compare the limitations and feasibility of these treatments.

例 12 和例 13 机器翻译版本确有语病,连接语叠加的问题一目了然。例 12 表转折关系的 although 和 yet 应删除一个,例 13 表因果关系的 because 和 so 保留一个就足够了。有趣的是,删除了冗余连接语的机器翻译仍然存在其他的冗余问题,仍需加工。例 12 的副词冗余表现为 still debatable,形容词冗余表现为 proven and well-tolerated,去除赘言后,例 12 可修改为:

例 12 译文修改为:Although it is debatable as to whether non-invasive respiratory support is the best option for acute respiratory failure, there is no denying that high-flow nasal cannula(HFNC)has been proven as a well-tolerated respiratory support technique in a variety of clinical settings.

形容词冗余也出现在例 13 中,用 normal 一词来修饰 OPN regulation 其实并无必要,英文译文可改为：

例 13 译文修改为：Because it interferes with OPN regulation, the blocking or silencing of OPN may also lead to other serious adverse effects, further research is needed to systematically compare the limitations and feasibility of these treatments.

除了英汉语言差异导致的误用和冗余,滥用连接词也是新手作者的通病之一。学习者在长久的应试训练下,刻意追求包括连接语在内的所谓"高级词汇",不仅段首要保证出现连接语,段落内也频繁使用连接语,如下例：

例 14：In addition to optimized synchronization, a controllable phase angle is also accomplished by UPSM. In phasor transformer based CSC, a controlled phase is indispensable for parallel systems to achieve reactive current control. Therefore, the proposed PSM allows a parallel single-stage resonant inverter to implement an advanced CSC algorithm. On the other hand, compared with two-stage resonant inverter, the proposed modulation and control scheme offers the same control capability in a single-stage resonant inverter with the simpler power circuit, hence, lower costs and higher efficiency are achieved. Meanwhile, a single-stage resonant inverter can provide better dynamic performance than a two-stage resonant inverter, so UPSM combined with a single-stage resonant inverter would be an optimal implementation of a high frequency power source.

在这个段落中,作者使用了七次连接语,试图强化句间的逻辑联系。然而,事与愿违,超量使用不仅不能帮助行文流畅,反而使表达显得生硬,干扰阅读。本句改写如下：

例 14 修改为：In addition to optimized synchronization, a controllable phase angle is also accomplished by UPSM. In phasor transformer based CSC, a controlled phase is indispensable for a parallel system to achieve reactive current control, which enables the parallel single-stage resonant inverter to implement an advanced CSC algorithm in the proposed PSM. However, compared with the two-stage resonant inverter, the proposed modulation and control scheme offers the same control capability in single-stage resonant inverter with the simpler power circuit, resulting in lower cost and higher efficiency. The single-stage resonant inverter can also provide better dynamic performance than two-stage resonant inverter. This means UPSM combined with single-stage resonant inverter would be an optimal implementation of high frequency power source.

3.2.3 范畴词的省略

英汉术语构成方式的差异可能导致汉语作者在用英语写作时将母语习惯迁移代

入,范畴词的使用就是其中一例。范畴词是指汉语命名中倾向于加范畴的词语,如问题、状态、主义、条件、能力、程度、情况、工作,有时本身没有实质意义,不需寻求英语对等词;同时,当英语术语为抽象名词时,本身即可具备汉语中"意义中心词＋范畴词"组合的意义和语法功能,此时加上范畴词无异于画蛇添足。

例如,"多糖酶水平升高"表达为 elevated polyase level 并非不可,但这个词组里的范畴词"水平"即使在汉语写作时也可以略去不用,词组简化为"多糖酶升高",可译为 elevated polyase、polyase elevation、polyase elevated 等。

某些术语更有约定俗成的表达,不仅不需要范畴词,连核心词汇也与汉语大相径庭,例如"细菌菌落现象"不应表达为 bacterial colony phenomenon,而应为 satellitism。

例 15:对肝脏再生的刺激作用

its stimulation ~~effect~~ to liver regeneration

此处范畴词 effect 可去除,下同。

例 16:检测增殖相关分子 Cyclin D1 和 Ki-67 的表达水平

detecting the expression ~~levels~~ of proliferation-related molecules Cyclin D1 and Ki-67

例 17:针对密切接触者的身份追踪及其隐私保护问题,本文进行了研究。

This paper examines the identity-tracking and privacy protection ~~issues~~ of the close-contacts.

例 18:结果表明,化合物对 UGM 具有较强的抑制作用。

Taken together, these results revealed that the compound provides a substantial inhibition ~~effect~~ on UGM.

归纳来看,英语医学写作并不是刻板和枯燥的,正确措辞不仅可以清楚地达意,也可使篇章逻辑更加清晰,行文简洁优美,更利于为编辑、审稿人和读者所接受,达成学术交流的目的。

第四节　练习巩固

1. 请把下面表格中缺失的术语或普通词填补完整。

	Terminologies(术语)	Plain words(普通词)
脱发	alopecia	
低血压		low blood pressure
百日咳		whooping cough
伤口	leision	
血栓	thrombosis	

	Terminologies（术语）	Plain words（普通词）
肝癌		liver tumor
硬化		hardening
黏膜	mucosa	

2. 观察下列句子,运用恰当的方法为画线的重复词汇进行同义替换。

（1）There is no current consensus regarding the most appropriate <u>treatment</u> for these patients，therefore this study intends to analyze the variables meaningful to <u>treatment</u> outcomes.

（2）Ferroptosis inducers have shown considerable effectiveness <u>in killing tumour cells</u> *in vitro*，yet there has been no obvious success <u>in killing tumour cells</u> in experimental animal models.

（3）Of the participants with <u>gonorrhea</u> culture available, tetracycline-resistant <u>gonorrhea</u> occurred in 5 of 13 in the doxycycline groups and 2 of 16 in the standard-care groups.

（4）However，it is <u>unclear</u> how stable these dynamic changes are，and it is <u>unclear</u> whether or not these dynamic changes provide significant insight into the underlying pathogenesis of asthma in these patients.

（5）A meta-analysis <u>published</u> in 2017 showed that two cups of coffee per day could reduce risk of hepatocellular carcinoma by 35%，but the mechanisms underlying the protective effects of coffee were not <u>published</u> in recent years.

3. 阅读下面的汉语句子,检查其译文,找出译文中用词冗余的问题,作出适当的修改,使译文简洁。

（1）近年来,非酒精性脂肪性肝炎研究领域已经取得相当多的进展。

In recent years，considerable progress has been made in the field of nonalcoholic steatohepatitis.

（2）目前缺少有效治疗药物和关键有效靶标。

There is a lack of effective therapeutic drugs and key effective targets.

（3）该病毒感染的临床表现差异大,包括无症状、感染性休克和多器官功能障碍等。

The clinical manifestations of this viral infection vary widely，ranging from asymptomatic，septic shock，to multiple organ dysfunction and so on.

（4）已经开发了几个模型和评分标准来评价肝功能储备,作为儿童患者生存的独立预后因素。

Several models and scoring criteria have been developed to evaluate liver function reserve as an independent prognostic factor for survival in pediatric patients.

第二章　名词化结构

第一节　引言

1.1　定义

　　名词化是指把句子中的动词或形容词转化成名词或名词词组,从而使名词或名词词组获得动词或形容词的意义而具有名词的语法功能。名词化是学术英语语篇中最普遍的特点之一。

　　医学写作是以事实为基础记述客观事物的,要求用词简洁、表达确切、结构严密、描述客观。如果句子的谓语动词加以名词化变形,并将其与主语或宾语加以整合,则实际起到了用名词性短语表达句子的作用,可使句子结构言简意赅,内部组织严密,并可以把更多的信息结构融于一体,使彼此的逻辑关系更明确,表达更细密,因而医学英语语篇写作青睐名词化结构。尽管如此,过量使用名词化结构极易造成冗余和行文僵化,不利于传达信息,应予以注意。

1.2　形式

　　名词化结构的形式相对简单,相应的动词或形容词变成名词,之后往往紧跟介词+名词/名词词组,构成名词性词组,例如:graying and loss of hair,在这个名词化结构中,动名词 graying 由形容词 gray 变来,名词 loss 由动词 lose 变来,之后紧跟 of+ hair(名词)。

　　英语作为典型的屈折语,词性变化一般要体现为形态变化:名词性词缀、动名词符号-ing 常用来构成名词化结构,如动词 enter,既可以加上-ance 变为 entrance,也可以变为动名词 entering;少数单词既具有动词属性也具有名词属性,则无须形态变化,例如 change、murder、protest 等。

1.3 类别

名词化结构主要分为两种：动词名词化结构和形容词名词化结构。如：loss of teeth、availability of health service，名词 loss 由动词 lose 变来，名词 availability 由形容词 available 变来。请看下面两个表格的内容。

Verb → Noun		Adjective → Noun	
demonstrate	demonstration	different	difference
inject	injection	valuable	value
identify	identification	active	activation
use	usage	appropriate	appropriateness
diagnose	diagnosis	absent	absence

1.4 作用

名词化结构在医学英语中出现频繁。它们可以浓缩信息，使语篇句子结构变得更加简洁（conciseness）；它们的使用，使语篇句子结构呈现多样性（variety）；名词化结构中过程参与者的隐去，使语篇语气增加客观性（objectivity）；名词化结构的使用，使句子表达紧凑严密，增加语篇句子准确性（preciseness）和逻辑性（logic）（详见第二节举例说明）；名词化结构的使用，使语篇句子实现前后连贯，提高语篇衔接性（coherence）。医学英语写作中正确使用名词化结构有助于提高医学英语写作的水平和质量。例如：

Sentences without nominalization	Sentences with nominalization
Influenza cases are rapidly increasing, which is causing concern for public health officials.	**The rapid increase** of influenza cases is causing concern for public health officials.
The hair is gray, the teeth are lost and the skin is wrinkled, which are the obvious characteristics of aging.	**Graying** of hair, **loss** of teeth, and **wrinkling** of skin are the obvious characteristics of aging.
ATP levels are required to be measured and subsequently established by a luminometer.	A luminometer is required for **measurement** and **subsequent establishment** of ATP levels.

第二节 举例说明

2.1 动词名词化结构

例 1：The **accumulation** of soluble and insoluble aggregated amyloid-beta（Aβ）may initiate or potentiate pathologic processes in Alzheimer's disease.

可溶性和不可溶性聚集性淀粉样蛋白（Aβ）的**积累**可能启动或增强阿尔茨海默病的病理过程。

例 2：However, the results of some studies have suggested that the **discontinuation** of RAS inhibitors in patients with advanced chronic kidney disease may increase the estimated glomerular filtration rate（eGFR）or slow its decline.

然而，一些研究结果提示，晚期慢性肾病患者**停用** RAS 抑制剂可能会升高肾小球滤过率（eGFR）估算值或减缓其降低。

例 3：The schematic shows **segmentation** of four cerebrum tissue volumes, followed by **estimation** of univariate centile scores, leading to the orthogonal **projection** of a single participant's scan（Subx）onto the four respective principal components of the CN（coloured axes and arrows）.

示意图显示了大脑四种组织的体积**分割**，然后**估计**单变量百分位数分数，从而将单个受试者的扫描（Subx）正交**投影**到 CN（彩色轴和箭头）的四个相应主成分上。

例 4：A neuropathological **examination** of brain tissue from 20 patients who died of the global pandemic showed infarcts in six patients, with most of these described as "small and patchy peripheral and deep parenchymal ischaemic infarcts," with no histological evidence of vasculitis reported.

20 例死于全球大流行病的患者脑组织神经病理学**检查**结果显示 6 例有梗死，其中大多数被描述为"小的片状的外周和深部实质缺血性梗死"，未有血管炎的组织学证据报告。

2.2 形容词名词化结构

例 5：This approach is conceptually similar to quantile rank mapping, as previously reported, where the **typicality** or **atypicality** of each phenotype in each scan is quantified by its score on the distribution of phenotypic parameters in the normative or reference sample of scans, with more atypical phenotypes having more extreme centile（or quantile）scores.

如前所述,这种方法在概念上类似于分位数秩映射,其中,每次扫描中各表型的**典型性**或**非典型性**通过其在扫描的规范样本或参考样本中表型参数**分布**的评分来量化:表型的非典型性越高,其百分位数(或分位数)值越极端。

例 6:Another case report of a patient with the epidemic disease and retiform purpura, a vasculitis mimic, clearly showed extensive cutaneous vascular thrombosis, an **absence** of inflammatory cells, and expression of terminal complement components in the vessel walls, further supporting complement pathway activation secondary to ischaemia.

另一例患有流行病合并网状紫癜(一种类似血管炎的疾病)的患者,其病例报告清楚显示,大面积皮肤血管血栓形成,炎症细胞**缺乏**,血管壁中出现终末补体成分,进一步支持了局部缺血后的补体通路活化。

例 7:Nevertheless, the hazard ratios for the cardiovascular outcomes were consistent with the **totality** of the evidence to date: a meta analysis showed that SGLT2 inhibitors lowered the risk of death from cardiovascular causes by 14% and lowered the risk of hospitalization for heart failure or death from cardiovascular causes by 23%.

然而,心血管疾病结局的风险比与迄今研究结果的**全部**证据一致:一项荟萃分析表明,SGLT2 抑制剂使心血管原因死亡风险降低了 14%,使心力衰竭住院或心血管原因死亡风险降低了 23%。

例 8:This approval was based on the results of the current Progress in Dermatomyositis (ProDERM) trial, which aimed to evaluate the **efficacy** and **safety** of this IVIG preparation in adults with dermatomyositis.

此次批准基于当前皮肌炎进展(ProDERM)试验的结果,该试验旨在评估 IVIG 制剂在成人皮肌炎患者中的**有效性**和**安全性**。

第三节　错例分析

例 1:To compare adverse event rates directly with those of other studies is challenging and warrants to consider several caveats.

直接比较本研究中不良事件发生率与其他研究中不良事件发生率具有挑战性,需要考虑几个注意事项。

分析:本句使用不定式短语 to compare adverse event rates directly with those of other studies 作为主语,尽管可以表意,但与 and 后面的信息有所脱节,在医学论文写作行文上显得松散,不够正式、简洁、严密。根据句子逻辑关系,可以考虑把动词 compare 和 consider 名词化,变成 comparison of 和 consideration of,使句子更紧凑严密。

改为：Direct comparison of adverse event rates with those of other studies is challenging and warrants consideration of several caveats.

例 2：Adverse events, serious adverse events, and fatalities were documented throughout the trial at each visit (scheduled or unscheduled) and up to 4 weeks after the IVIG or placebo was last administrated. Trial investigators assessed the causal adverse events that occurred at their site.

在整个试验过程中，分别记录了每次就医（计划或非计划的）以及最后一次 IVIG 或安慰剂给药后 4 周的不良事件、严重不良事件和死亡事件。试验研究人员评估了在试验现场发生的不良事件的因果关系。

分析：本句使用了时间状语从句 after the IVIG or placebo was last administrated，从句中强调的是主语所指的事物 IVIG or placebo，根据句子上下文，强调的应该是给药的时间，可以利用动词名词化结构使前后时间紧密关联，即把 last administrated 变成动名词结构 last administration of。另外，在最后一句中，动词 assessed 评估的对象应该是因果关系，而不是 adverse events，所以需要把形容词 causal 变成相应的名词 causality of。

改为：Adverse events, serious adverse events, and fatalities were documented throughout the trial at each visit (scheduled or unscheduled) and up to 4 weeks after the last administration of IVIG or placebo. Trial investigators assessed the causality of adverse events that occurred at their site.

例 3：The strategies used in cognitive therapy focus on helping the patient to discover their implicit or explicit dysfunctional beliefs about sleep, gathering evidence to decide whether these beliefs are valid and generating responses to cope with or overcome them.

认知疗法的策略主要是帮助患者找出其或隐性或显性的睡眠功能失调性观念，收集支持或反对这些观念的证据，并引导患者做出反应，应对或克服这些观念。

分析：本句看似较长，其实结构简单，谓语 focus on 后面的宾语是呈平行结构的三个并列词组，且三个词组都是动名词词组。然而细看之下可以发现，第二个宾语 gathering evidence to decide whether these beliefs are valid，使得该宾语中嵌套了从句，与前后两个宾语不平衡。通过名词化变形可以减掉这一从句，实现完美的平行并列。

改为：The strategies used in cognitive therapy focus on helping the patients to discover their implicit or explicit dysfunctional beliefs about sleep, gathering evidence for and against the validity of these beliefs, and generating responses to cope with or overcome them.

例 4：Taken together, identifying this sperm-specific ribosome, we should greatly and expansively understand ribosome and regulate the tissue-specific protein expression pattern in mammals.

总而言之，鉴别出这种精子的特异性核糖体，将大大增加我们对核糖体功能以及哺乳动物蛋白的表达模式组织特异性调节的认识。

分析：本句中现在分词短语 identifying this sperm-specific ribosome 作为非谓语成分，表示伴随状况，主句中人称代词 we 作为动作执行者，显得主观，可信度不高。根据分析前后两部分句意的逻辑关系，前后两部分存在前因后果的关系。在医学论文写作中，为了使前后句子更加紧凑及句式更加多样化，可以考虑使用动词名词化结构把前后两部分句子整合成一个完整的句子。

改为：Taken together, identifcation of this sperm-specific ribosome should greatly expand our understanding of ribosome function and tissue-specific regulation of protein expression pattern in mammals.

第四节　练习巩固

1. 请把下面表格中的动词或形容词变成相应的名词。

Verb	→	Noun	Adjective	→	Noun
use			present		
express			specific		
inhibit			effective		
clear			safe		
analyze			typical		
study			accurate		
exam			wide		
detect			deep		

2. 请将下列句子中的名词化结构用下划线画出来。

（1）A randomized, placebo-controlled trial involving 15 patients and several noncontrolled studies have suggested that IVIG may be effective in the treatment of dermatomyositis.

（2）The authors vouch for the accuracy and completeness of the data and the reporting of adverse events and for the fidelity of the trial to the protocol, available with the full text of this article at NEJM. org.

(3) A sensitivity analysis of the primary end point was performed with the use of a logistic-regression model that included the PhGA disease-activity score as a covariate.

(4) The widths of 95% confidence intervals for the between-group differences in the secondary end-point analyses were not adjusted for multiple comparisons, and no definite conclusions can be drawn from these data.

(5) The mechanism of action of IVIG in patients with dermatomyositis is not understood but may involve inhibition of complement consumption and interference with formation of the membrane attack complex.

(6) In addition, IVIG may lead to down-regulation of cytokines and chemokines and modification of gene expression in patients with dermatomyositis.

(7) For missing measurements of body weight, the last available body weight was used for all calculations related to dosing.

3. 请把下面的中文句子翻译成英文,黑体词语请使用名词化结构。

(1) **过量进食**还与进餐时间和代谢的内源性昼夜(circadian)节律紊乱有关。

_____

(2) 我们去除具有较低读取意义(low read depth)的波峰值,以避免节律性染色质开放的假阳性**检测**。

_____

(3) 免疫分析显示 CAR T 细胞仅在肿瘤内**扩增**,激活标志物增加,耗竭标志物减少。

_____

(4) 此外,对两种抗原输入(CAR 和 synNotch 抗原)的**识别**将进一步增强肿瘤靶向的特异性。

_____

(5) 重要的是,这些平台在研究 SARS-CoV-2 感染方面的**相关性**已经得到证明。

_____

第三章　平行结构

第一节　引言

1.1　定义

在英语语法中,平行结构(Parallelism)是指两个或两个以上密切相关单词、短语或从句具有相似的语法结构或句法模式。通常,这些单词、短语或从句以相同的并列语法形式出现,如一个名词与其他名词并列,一个形容词与其他形容词并列,一个-ing形式与其他-ing形式并列,一个不定式短语与其他不定式短语并列,一个被动语态句子与其他被动语态句子并列等等。

平行结构是表达复杂概念的一种有效方法,能使复杂的文本更易于阅读、理解和记忆。工整的结构,能使语言表达简洁明晰,并突出重点内容,使文句铿锵有力,层次清晰,意思脉络分明。平行结构特征符合科技英语语篇的要求,是科技英语语篇中最普遍的特点之一。

医学英语写作是以事实为基础记述客观事物,需要把专业深奥的复杂信息有效表达出来,因而医学英语写作也青睐平行结构。

1.2　形式

根据平行结构的定义,平行结构的形式不固定,非常灵活。在符合英语语法的要求下,根据写作需要可以选择不同的形式,可以是名词的并列、动词的并列、形容词的并列、介词短语的并列、名词短语的并列、分词短语的并列、主动语态句子的并列、被动语态句子的并列等等。在有平行结构的句子中,平行成分间通常会有多个逗号(,),通常会用连词"and"来连接最后一个并列成分。

1.3　类别

根据平行结构的定义,平行结构主要分为三种类型:单词平行、短语平行、句子平行。

类别	例子
单词平行	**Sustainable，scaled，**and **global** manufacturing would improve the response to future pandemics.（形容词平行）
短语平行	These strategies should consider variations in **available financing，service delivery，public health infrastructure，disease burden，vaccine acceptance，**and other factors across countries.（名词短语平行）
句子平行	In the systematic section，**the normal structure and function of each organ is summarized，the pathological basis for clinical signs and symptoms is described，**and **the clinical implications of each disease are emphasized.**（被动语态句子平行）

第二节　举例说明

2.1　单词平行

例 1：Global health funders and governments should **require** and **prioritize** digital infrastructure to **deliver，track，**and **measure** the impact of adult vaccines，injectables，and other interventions.（动词平行）

全球卫生资助者和政府应**要求**并**优先考虑**数字基础设施，以**提供、跟踪和测量**成人疫苗、注射剂和其他干预措施的影响。

例 2：In the adult vaccine space，new products at multiple stages of preclinical and clinical development for **coronaviruses，influenza，**and **RSV**（respiratory syncytial virus）are expected to emerge in the coming months and years.（名词平行）

在成人疫苗领域，针对**冠状病毒、流感病毒和呼吸道合胞病毒**（RSV），处于临床前和临床开发多个阶段的新产品，预计将在未来几个月和几年内问世。

例 3：Sometimes，more detailed data may need to be collected and analyzed to determine whether health services are **available，accessible，effective，**and **efficient.**（形容词平行）

有时，可能需要收集和分析更详细的数据，以确定健康服务是否**可用、可获得**，以及是否**有效和高效**。

例 4：A global adult disease prevention programme，supported by **geographically** distributed manufacturing and **digitally** enabled cold chain，service delivery，and recording，could have profound implications for health worldwide between disease outbreaks and also create the systems to respond to future pathogen threats.

有了**地理性**分布制造和**电子化**冷链、服务交付和记录的支持，全球成人疾病预防规划可以对疾病暴发期的全球卫生健康产生深远影响，也可以创建多种系统以应对未来

的病原体威胁。（副词平行）

2.2 短语平行

例 5：The pandemic highlighted the role of community-based and primary care sites **to deliver vaccines** and **to build reliable cold chains**. （不定式短语并列）

大流行凸显了社区和初级保健站在**运送疫苗**和**建立可靠冷链**方面的作用。

例 6：**The reported incidences of** the epidemic disease breakthrough infection and **the reported development of** active virus in previously vaccinated individuals，range from 0. 4% to 9. 5%，depending on the vaccine type，the time elapsed after vaccination，the percentage of vaccinated people，and viral variants.

根据疫苗类型、接种疫苗后的时间、接种疫苗的人数百分比和病毒变体的不同，报告的流行病突破**感染率**和以前接种过疫苗的个人活跃病毒发展的**发生率**从 0.4%到 9.5%不等。

例 7：The word epidemiology comes from the Greek words *epi*，**meaning** on or upon，*demos*，**meaning** people，and *logos*，**meaning** the study of. （现在分词短语平行）

流行病学这个词来自希腊语 *epi*，**意思是关于**；*demos*，**意思是人**；*logos*，**意思是研究**。

例 8：**For adults with diabetes and hypertension**，clinical practice guidelines support an SBP goal of less than 130 mm Hg. **For adults with chronic kidney disease**，the most recent *Kidney Disease：Improving Global Outcomes* guidelines recommended an SBP goal of less than 120 mm Hg when tolerated，but other guidelines recommend an SBP goal of less than 130mmHg. （介词短语平行）

对于**患有糖尿病和高血压的成人**，临床实践指南支持将收缩压目标值定在低于 130 毫米汞柱以下。对于**患有慢性肾脏疾病的成人**，最新的《肾脏疾病：改善全球结局》指南建议，在可以耐受情况下，收缩压目标值应低于 120 毫米汞柱，但其他指南建议收缩压目标值应低于 130 毫米汞柱。

2.3 句子平行

例 9：Based on self-reported data from a survey of hypertension prevalence in 533,306 adults，it was estimated that **eliminating hypertension in women would reduce population mortality by approximately 7. 3% compared with 0. 1% for hyperlipidemia，4. 1% for diabetes，4. 4% for cigarette smoking，and 1. 7% for obesity. Eliminating hypertension in men would reduce population mortality by approximately 3. 8% compared with 2. 0% for hyperlipidemia，1. 7% for diabetes，5. 1% for cigarette smoking，and 2. 6% for obesity.** （主谓宾结构句子平行）

对 533,306 名成年人高血压患病率调查的自我报告数据显示，消除女性高血压可使人口死亡率降低约 7.3%,而消除高脂血症、消除糖尿病、停止吸烟和消除肥胖可使人口死亡率分别降低 0.1%、4.1%、4.4%和 1.7%。消除男性高血压可使人口死亡率降低约 3.8%,而消除高脂血症、消除糖尿病、戒烟和消除肥胖可使人口死亡率分别降低 2.0%、1.7%、5.1%和 2.6%。

例 10:Measuring **what matters most to young people and their families** and **what leads to optimal interpersonal, educational, and occupational outcomes,** are important considerations for deciding which interventions provide the most benefit for patients, families, and society.(特殊疑问词引导的句子平行)

衡量什么对年轻人和他们的家庭最重要,衡量什么会带来最佳的人际关系、教育和职业结果,这些是非常重要的考虑因素,决定了哪些干预措施会给患者、家庭和社会带来最大益处。

第三节　错例分析

例 1:Depression is a leading contributor to the global burden of disease and is associated with personal, societal, and economy burden.

抑郁症是造成全球疾病负担的主要因素,与个体、社会和经济负担有关。

分析:通读此句,句子明显存在单词平行结构。根据上下文及连词"and",可以看出是 personal、societal 和 economy 三个词平行,但是句中 economy 是名词,不能与前面两个形容词平行,应该改为"economic"。

改为:Depression is a leading contributor to the global burden of disease and is associated with personal, societal, and economic burden.

例 2:Depression in young people is an increasing concern not only because it occurs during a period of rapid social, emotional, and cognitive development, and key life transitions, but also its prevalence in young people (ie, ages 10—24 years) has risen sharply in the past decade, especially in females.

青少年抑郁症日益受到关注,这不仅是因为青少年正处于社会、情感和认知的快速发展期以及人生的关键转折期,而且在过去十年中,青少年(即 10—24 岁)抑郁症的发病率急剧上升,尤其是女性。

分析:通读此句,句中明显存在单词平行和句子平行结构。单词平行是 3 个形容词 social、emotional 和 cognitive 的平行。句子平行,根据句子前后逻辑关系和英语短语结构,可以看出是 not only ... but also ... 结构,not only 后跟了 because 引导的原因从句,根据平行结构的定义,but also 后面也同样跟了 because 引导的原因从句,但原句中没有,所以需要加上 because,变成... **but also because** its prevalence in young people ... 。

改为：Depression in young people is an increasing concern <u>not only because</u> it occurs during a period of rapid social, emotional, and cognitive development, and key life transitions, <u>but also because</u> its prevalence in young people (ie, ages 10—24 years) has risen sharply in the past decade, especially in females.

例 3：Eating patterns associated with lowering dietary sodium intake include eating fresh rather than processed foods, reducing portion size, avoiding foods especially high in sodium content, to read food labels for packaged and prepared foods, choosing condiments and seasonings with low sodium content, and to attempt sodium substitutions by using herbs, spices, or potassium-enriched salt substitutes.

与降低钠摄入量相关的饮食模式包括：食用新鲜食品而不是加工食品，减少分量，避免钠含量特别高的食物，阅读包装食品和预制食品的食品标签，选择低钠含量的调味品和调味料，并尝试使用草药、香料或富含钾的盐替代品来替代钠。

分析：通读此句，句中明显存在短语平行结构。尽管句子很长，但通过逗号（,）分析句子结构，可以看出句子谓语动词 include（及物动词）后面需要跟名词或动名词（V+ing），但可以看出句中 V+ing 和 to+do 混杂，前后不一致，需要调整为统一的 V+ing 形式，构成对等的平行结构。因此，原句中 to read 需要改为 reading，to attempt 需要改为 attempting。

改为：Eating patterns associated with lowering dietary sodium intake include <u>eating</u> fresh rather than processed foods, <u>reducing</u> portion size, <u>avoiding</u> foods especially high in sodium content, <u>reading</u> food labels for packaged and prepared foods, <u>choosing</u> condiments and seasonings with low sodium content, <u>and attempting</u> sodium substitutions by using herbs, spices, or potassium-enriched salt substitutes.

例 4：This finding suggests that if hospitals had data that were more reliable and more routinely collected, it is possible that monitoring could be improved, adverse event rates would be reduced, and improvement strategies could be shared through careful study of interventions.

这项发现表明，如果医院拥有更可靠且更常规的数据收集，监测工作可能会得到改善，不良事件率将会降低，并且通过对干预措施进行仔细研究可以共享改进策略。

分析：通读此句，句中明显存在句子平行结构。根据逗号的连续使用和连词 and，可以看出后半部分句子中存在句子平行结构：主语＋could be＋过去分词（V-ed）。后半部分 that 从句中三个分句的结构是 could be improved、would be reduced、could be shared，显而易见，would be reduced 与其前后的 could be ＋V-ed 不一致不对等。因此，需要把 would be reduced 更改为 could be reduced，与其前后构成行文上的平行结构。

改为：This finding suggests that if hospitals had data that were more reliable and more routinely collected, it is possible that monitoring <u>could be improved</u>, adverse event rates <u>could be reduced</u>, and improvement strategies <u>could be shared</u> through careful study of interventions.

第四节　练习巩固

1. 请将下列句子中的平行结构用下划线画出。

（1）The use of CO-RADS and CT severity scores is useful for the triage, diagnosis, and management decisions of patients presenting with possible epidemic at the emergency department.

（2）This review summarizes current evidence involving treatment of hypertension and emphasizing the 2017 ACC/AHA high BP guideline recommendations.

（3）Epidemiologic studies have repeatedly documented a progressive, direct, quantitative, dose-response relationship between alcohol consumption and level of BP, as well as the incidence of hypertension.

（4）First-line pharmacologic therapy for hypertension consists of thiazide diuretics, calcium channel blockers, and angiotensin-converting enzyme inhibitors or angiotensin receptor blockers, or available 2-drug combinations.

（5）Prevalence of depression is particularly high in people who have special educational needs or a chronic health problem, and in people who come from socioeconomically disadvantaged households.

2. 请根据上下文用括号中词语的正确形式补充完成下列句子。

（1）Established nonpharmacologic interventions for the prevention and _____ (treat) of hypertension are _____ (loss) weight, reducing dietary sodium, increasing potassium intake, _____ (consumption) a heart-healthy diet, engaging in physical activity, and reducing alcohol consumption.

（2）Which of the above-mentioned structured reporting systems to use or how to integrate them for patients care depends on the _____ (reproducible), _____ (reliable), and _____ (simple) of these reporting systems.

（3）The sponsor _____ (collect) the data, provided the IVIG and placebo, _____ (monitor) the conduct of the trial, and _____ (performance) the statistical analyses.

（4）"_____ (cure) sometimes, _____ (relieve) often, and _____ (comfort) always" is a French saying as apt today as it was five centuries ago—as is

Francis Peabody's admonition: "The secret of the care of the patient is in caring for the patient."

(5) This method not only _____ (enhance) treatment adherence and _____ (improve) treatment control but also helps to avoid overtreating white coat hypertension (BP high in the office but normal at home) and _____ (allow) detection of masked hypertension (BP normal in the office but high at home).

3. 请把下面的中文句子翻译成英文,注意务必使用平行结构。

(1) 流行病学是数据驱动的,依赖于系统和公正的方法来收集、分析和解释数据。

_____

_____

(2) 参与者以 1∶2 的比例被随机分配,要么接受单次结肠镜检查(受邀组),要么不接受邀请或检查(常规护理组)。

_____

_____

(3) 临床医学与病理学是相辅相成、不可分割的。如果不了解病理学,临床医学就无法开展;如果没有临床医学的背景就无法理解病理学。

_____

_____

(4) 流行病学的基本方法往往依赖于仔细观察和使用有效对照组,以评估所观察到的情况,例如在特定时期内特定地区的疾病病例数或患者接触疾病的频率,是否与预期的情况不同。

_____

_____

(5) 要评估人口或社区的健康状况,必须按人、地点和时间确定和分析相关数据来源。

_____

_____

第四章 省略结构

第一节 引言

1.1 定义

省略(Ellipsis)是为了避免重复,将句子中的某些成分省去的语言现象。在医学英语写作中非常常见,其目的是为了避免重复,突出新信息并使上下文紧密连接;同时,在文本中节约用词是一条重要的修辞原则。只要不损害语法结构或者因此产生歧义,能省略的就可以省略。英语表达中存在多种多样的省略,如能熟练地掌握其用法,弄清省略部分的含义,对医学英语的文献阅读也会有所裨益。

这里主要针对在医学英语写作中,作者受到汉语思维的影响,对于该不该省略、何时能省略等情况做简单叙述。

1.2 标准

在医学英语文本中出现的省略现象通常会符合下面的标准,读者在阅读中容易识别,一看便知:

(1) 被省略的部分是结构成分和含义相同的部分,且一目了然,容易还原;

(2) 被省略的部分还原后应该是语法结构正确的句子。

1.3 类别

省略有三种类型:语篇省略、语境省略和结构省略。我们在这里主要讨论医学英语写作中常见的语篇省略。

所谓语篇省略指能在上下文中找到先行项的省略结构。医学英语写作中,语篇省略主要体现在并列句和复合句中的不同成分省略。并列句中可以省略共同的主语或宾语;若主语不同而后面谓语相同,也可省略;若主谓成分都相同,则都可以省略;重复的介词、连词及后续部分也可以省略。复合句的省略在本章中着重讨论状语从句和定语从句,从句中会出现主谓成分、宾语、表语省略的现象;偶尔在 than 引导的比较状语从句中会出现省略主句的情况。

第二节　举例说明

2.1　并列句中的省略

例 1：Participants were categorized into the favourable group if they had four to six healthy lifestyle factors, (participants were categorized) into the average group for two to three (healthy lifestyle) factors, and (participants were categorized) into the unfavourable group for zero to one (healthy lifestyle) factor.

如果受试者具备四到六个健康生活方式因素，就被归入有利组，两到三个因素则被归入平均组，零到一个因素则归入不利组。

分析：本句中有三个并列句，主结构为 participants were categorized into ... if they had ... factors，表明根据健康生活方式因素的多少可被划分进特定组别。其中括号部分为省略成分，分别为主谓结构与定语成分，因为三句结构基本一致，语态一致，所以后两句中可以省略先行项中的两处相同结构（participants were categorized, healthy lifestyle）。省略后结构清楚，意思一目了然，读者也可以轻松还原。

例 2：Anxiety disorders have a lifetime prevalence of approximately 34% in the US, (anxiety disorders) are often chronic, and (anxiety disorders) significantly impair quality of life and functioning.

在美国，焦虑症的终生患病率约为 34%，通常是慢性的，并严重损害生活质量和功能。

分析：在本句的平行结构中，主语一致都是 anxiety disorders，故后两个并列句中的主语都可以省略，这样显得行文简洁紧凑。

例 3：Up to 71% to 97.8% of patients with anxiety disorders are not correctly diagnosed and approximately 41% (of patients) are not treated.

高达 71% 至 97.8% 的焦虑症患者没有得到正确诊断，约 41% 的患者没有得到治疗。

分析：本句中先行项为 of patients，所以并列句中百分比后省略了 of patients。

例 4：Panic attacks may occur in response to specific stressful events or (occur) as part of any anxiety disorder.

恐慌发作可能是对特定压力事件的反应，也可能是任何焦虑症的一部分。

分析：本句可以看作平行结构中谓语的省略，其中先行项为 occur，所以 or 之后省略了 occur。

例 5：Fertility preservation with （hormonal stimulation） or without hormonal stimulation was not statistically significantly associated with any increased risk of relapse or death from breast cancer in this population-based Swedish cohort study.

在这项基于人群的瑞典队列研究中,通过（激素刺激）或不通过激素刺激来保持生育能力与乳腺癌复发或死亡风险增加在统计学上没有明显关联。

分析:本句主语 fertility preservation 的并列后置定语由两个介词短语 with or without ... 组成,其中名词成分相同,故不用重复两遍。

2.2 复合句中的省略

例 6：Although the risk of the in-hospital composite outcome was also significantly reduced with nirmatrelvir plus ritonavir use compared with non-use （of nirmatrelvir plus ritonavir）, this reduction was mainly driven by a substantial mortality benefit rather than reducing IMV initiation or ICU admission.

尽管与不使用相比,使用尼马特雷韦加利托那韦也显著降低了院内综合结果的风险,这一下降主要是由显著的死亡率效益推动的,与减少 IMV 的发生或 ICU 入院无关。

分析:这里的省略出现在让步状语从句中,特定药物使用与否并非是造成结果的主要原因,在从句的比较概念中药物名称不用再次提及,可以省略。

例 7：Hypercalcemia is defined by a serum calcium value above the upper limit of the normal range, （which is） defined as greater than 2 SDs above the population mean.

高钙血症定义为血清钙值高于正常范围的上限,即高于总体均值 2 个标准差。

分析:本句中主句在逗号之后应当是一个非限制性定语从句,其中 which is 不影响句子意思的体现,故可以省略。

在 when、while、if、as、though （although）、whether 等引导的时间、条件、方式、让步状语中,如果谓语动词是 be,而且其主语跟主句的主语相同或为 it 时,从句的主语和 be 动词就可以省略。

例 8：Many patients developed empyemas as a complication of parenchymal diseases, frequently while （they were） on antimicrobial therapy.

多数间质性病变者并发脓胸,这种情况常见于抗菌属治疗过程中。

分析:本句从句中的主语 they 指代主句中的 many patients,主从句中主语一致,谓语动词是 were,故可以省略。

例 9：In patients with a systolic blood pressure of at least 90 mmHg, the following 3 steps can be used to evaluate a patient with possible PE: assessment of the clinical probability of PE, D-dimer testing if (it is) indicated, and chest imaging if (it is) indicated.

在收缩压至少为 90 毫米汞柱的患者中，以下 3 个步骤可用于评估可能患有 PE 的患者：评估 PE 的临床概率，如果需要，可进行 D-二聚体检测以及胸部成像。

分析：上句画线部分被省略，原因在于句子提示评估的三步骤中后两种都包含了同样的一个条件句，其中的主谓结构 it is 没有实际意义，可以省略。括号中显示还原的内容，还原后语法结构正确。

2.3 不适用省略的情况

例 10：Hypercalcemia affects approximately 1% of the general population and approximately 2% of patients with cancer.

高钙血症影响约 1% 的普通人群和约 2% 的癌症患者。

分析：上句中出现的两个并列的宾语中虽然都有百分比数字（1%、2%），但指示了后面两类不同人群，所以不能使用省略原则。

例 11：Of 7 533 identified articles, 98 (articles) were included, consisting of 13 randomized clinical trials (RCTs), 4 meta-analyses, 17 longitudinal studies, 14 cross-sectional studies, 29 case reports/case series, and 21 reviews.

在 7 533 篇已确定的文章中，收录了 98 篇相关文章，包括 13 项随机临床试验（RCTs）、4 项 meta 分析、17 项纵向研究、14 项横断面研究、29 篇病例报告/病例系列和 21 篇综述。

分析：本句只省略了数字 98 之后的 articles，而后面的数字表示不同类型研究方法的文章数量，所以不可使用省略原则。

第三节 错例分析

例 1：Subsequent attempts to block this molecule in patients with alcohol associated hepatitis were unsuccessful and associated with severe and life-threatening infections, probably due to its role in liver regeneration and protection against bacterial infections.

随后，有人试图阻断酒精相关性肝炎患者体内的该分子，但没有成功，而且还引发了严重的、危及生命的感染，这可能是由于其在肝脏再生和预防细菌感染中起了作用。

分析：此句中平行结构左边是系表结构，右边是被动语态，虽然都有 be 动词，但是语法结构不同，语义也不一致，故不能省略，因为省去的词，不仅需要形态相同，而且功能也应相同。

改为：Subsequent attempts to block this molecule in patients with alcohol associated hepatitis were unsuccessful and <u>were associated</u> with …

例 2：The chordaetendineae of the left ventricle of 200 normal hearts of adults were studied and the classification of the chordae discussed.

本文对 200 例成人正常心脏的左心室的腱索做了观察，并对腱索的分类做了探讨。

分析：首先，"本文探讨"需用现在时，"观察腱索"用过去时，因此本句前后两个并列句时态不同，不同时态和不同属的助动词是不能省略的。

改为：The chordae tendineae of the left ventricle of 200 normal hearts of adults were studied and the classification of the chordae <u>is</u> discussed.

例 3：Parents or teachers may notice that a child has trouble with ADHD symptoms and needs to be evaluated to see if they have the disorder, so healthcare providers <u>may offer to evaluate or refer</u> the child to a specialist.

父母或老师可能会注意到孩子有多动症的症状，需要进行评估以查看他们是否患有这种疾病，医务人员可能会提供评估或将孩子转诊给专家。

分析：本句中有一个 or 引导的并列成分，从结构上看是谓语动词 offer 后两个不定式 to evaluate 和（to）refer the child … 的并列，那也就是说评估和转诊这两个动作都是医务人员可能提供的帮助；但是仔细从意义上看的话，会发现医务人员可以提供评估服务，也可以不评估而直接交给专家来判断。本句的并列成分并不适用省略原则，因为省略后改变了原结构和句意，不符合省略现象应遵循的标准。

改为：… healthcare providers may offer to evaluate or <u>may refer</u> the child to a specialist.

例 4：People with fluctuating weight, blood pressure, cholesterol and/or blood sugar levels are at higher risk of heart attack and stroke <u>than</u> with more stable readings.

体重、血压、胆固醇和/或血糖水平波动较大的人心脏病发作和中风的风险高于这些数值更稳定的人。

分析：本句比较的并非是数值，而是具备不同数值的主体（人），所以后者不应该省略主体。

改为：People with fluctuating weight, blood pressure, cholesterol and/or blood sugar levels are at higher risk of heart attack and stroke <u>than those/people</u> with more stable readings.

第四节　练习巩固

1. 请将下列句子译成英语。

（1）这些症状可能单独存在或成群存在，尽管它们的严重程度各不相同，但许多症状极大地影响了人们的健康和生活计划。

_____

_____

（2）这一变化旨在确定轻症酒精相关性肝炎的患者，有时这一疾病也被称为"非严重或中度酒精相关性肝炎"。

_____

_____

（3）事实上，最近的一项研究表明，尽管60％的提供者报告称将酒精使用障碍患者转诊做行为治疗，但71％的提供者从未开过药物治疗处方，因为他们不太愿意这样做。

_____

_____

（4）我们采用回顾性队列设计作为主要分析，病例对照设计作为敏感性分析。

_____

_____

2. 请将下列句子中的可省略部分用括号画出。

（1）HCC, biliary obstruction, or Budd-Chiari syndrome perform Doppler abdominal ultrasonography and, if it is indicated, CT or MRI-MRCPHCC.

（2）In patients at high risk of having bacterial meningitis, antibiotic therapy should be started promptly and continued while they are awaiting blood and CSF cultures.

（3）Adjunctive dexamethasone should be used in patients with bacterial meningitis but should be stopped if Listeria monocytogenes is confirmed.

（4）Among US youth who are aged 15 to 24 years, intentional self-harm is the second leading cause of death and it is accounted for 6807 deaths in 2018.

（5）The funder of the study had no role in study design, no role in data collection, no role in data analysis, or no role in data interpretation.

（6）The distribution of propensity scores in oral antiviral and matched control groups were highly overlapping, and it was indicating an acceptable quality of matching for our propensity-score models.

第五章 成分后移

第一节 引言

在医学英语论文中,我们会发现并不是所有句子都遵循正常的语序。如果句子的某个成分移出其正常位置,向后迁移,我们称这种现象为句子成分的后移(postposition)。这种语法机制通过改变词序,使相对较"重"即信息较多的成分出现在其规范位置的右侧,因此也称为"右移位"。语言学家认为后移是为了减少"中心嵌入结构",使英语句子易于解析。

后移是书面英语中常见的现象,有时是为了强调句子的某个成分而采取的强调手段之一,有时是为了使句子保持平衡以符合英语表达的语言习惯,有时则是为了语篇的展开和连贯性。下面我们来谈谈医学英语论文中常见的句子成分后移的几种情况。

第二节 举例说明

2.1 主语后移

英文句子的正常词序是主语在前,谓语在后,句首是主语的经典位置。但是,有时由于主语过长,为了遵循末端中心的原则而将主语后移(句首用 it、there 作形式主语),从而使句子的结构变得匀称。

例 1:It is advisable to perform AQP4-IgG testing before making a diagnosis of lupus myelitis.

建议在诊断狼疮性脊髓炎之前进行 AQP4-IgG 检测。

例 2:We recategorized other routes of administration as subcutaneous;however, it is possible that we erroneously recategorized vaccinations administered incorrectly.

我们将其他给药途径重归类为皮下给药;然而,对接种方式有误的情况有可能是分类不当。

例 3：To improve outcomes in hepatocellular carcinoma, it will be essential to decipher how key clinical and molecular characteristics influence disease course and treatment response.

为改善肝细胞癌的预后，破解关键的临床和分子特征如何影响病程和治疗反应至关重要。

以 it 作为句子的形式主语，还可以将字数更多，信息更复杂的结构后置。

例 4：It has been estimated that more than 10% of PD cases can be diagnosed incorrectly by movement disorder specialists when clinical signs are the only basis for diagnosis.

当临床症状作为唯一的诊断基础时，估计超过 10% 的帕金森病患者会被运动失调专家误诊。

例 5：Despite advances in slowing disease progression, there is no available treatment that depletes transthyretin amyloidosis from the heart for the amelioration of cardiac diseases.

尽管减缓疾病进展方面有些进步，但目前尚无疗法能够去除心脏转甲状腺素蛋白淀粉样变性以缓解心脏病。

2.2 定语后移

后移的定语有各种形式，以名词或名词性短语、不定式短语、分词短语以及从句为主。需要说明的是，医学论文包含的信息密度极高，因此句子的限定成分通常相当复杂，定语经常需要借助多种形式呈现，不仅需要后移，后移的定语往往多层嵌套。

例 6：We conducted a double-blind, randomized, placebo-controlled trial of oral metformin in adults who were hospitalized with obesity and had evidence of disrupted energy balance.

我们对因肥胖症住院且有能量平衡紊乱证据的成人进行了一项双盲、随机、安慰剂对照的口服二甲双胍试验。

现将常见的几种定语后移举例如下。

2.2.1 名词或名词性短语作定语时的后移

作为定语的词类除了形容词，还包括名词，然而，与汉语倾向于左向分支，将名词定语直接置于被修饰词前面的习惯不同，英语中相当比例的名词性定语需要借助介词，后移到中心词之后，常用的介词包括 of、with、on 等。

例 7：Currently available data on pregnant women indicate no malformative or fetal/neonatal toxicity.

目前可获得的孕妇数据显示没有畸形或胎儿/新生儿毒性。

例 8：The correct diagnosis of classical leptin deficiency or leptin dysfunction with inactive or antagonistic variants is a requisite for the personalized treatment of affected patients.

正确诊断经典瘦素缺乏症或瘦素功能障碍与非活性或拮抗变异体是决定患者个性化治疗的必要条件。

2.2.2 不定式短语作定语时的后移

例 9：The liver capacity was explained in the previous chapter to store carbohydrates as glycogen and to release glucose to maintain the normal concentration of glucose in the blood.

前章已解释了肝脏能以糖原形式储存糖，并能释放葡萄糖以保持血液中的葡萄糖含量正常。

例 10：The present plan is being undertaken to develop methods for recording and processing the fetal ECG obtained from maternal abdominal electrodes.

当前计划意欲建立从母体腹壁的电极获得胎儿心电图的记录及处理方法。

2.2.3 分词短语作定语时的后移

分词作定语包括现在分词与过去分词两种，现各举一例如下：

例 11：Artificial intelligence using computer-aided diagnosis (CADx) in real time with images acquired during colonoscopy may help colonoscopists distinguish between neoplastic polyps requiring removal and nonneoplastic polyps not requiring removal.

实时结合结肠镜检获得的图像，使用计算机辅助诊断（CADx）的人工智能可以帮助结肠镜检查医师区分需要切除的肿瘤性息肉和不需要切除的非肿瘤性息肉。

例 12：According to Traditional Chinese Medicine, the change in circulation produced by the hot bath has a beneficial effect in cases of stagnation of blood in the deeper organs of the body.

中医认为热水澡使血液循环发生变化，对于治疗身体深层器官的血液阻滞有积极的作用。

2.2.4 定语从句的后移

与英语句子中的其他定语成分一样，定语从句也位于被修饰的名词之后，因此可以说相对于汉语发生了从句位置的后移。

例 13：Data will be presented which suggests that sudden death ischemic heart disease may be due to hypomagnesemia in and around the coronary arterial and arteriolar vessels.

我们将报道由冠状动脉及周围血管低血镁引起缺血性心脏猝死的数据。

例 14：Early on in the patient's course，we contacted the pharmaceutical company that produces recombinant ADAMTS13 for emergency compassionate use.

在患者治疗早期，我们联系了生产重组 ADAMTS13 的制药公司，用于紧急治疗。

以上两句中出现的均为定语从句的后移，也是定语后移中最常见的一种情况。

需要注意的是，当中心词既有短语又有定语从句作后置定语时，一般的顺序是短语在前，从句在后。例如：

例 15：A patient is described with a 27-year-history of chronic relapsing Reiter's syndrome who developed secondary amyloidosis.

本文报道了一例有 27 年慢性复发性莱特尔氏综合征的患者发生继发性淀粉样病变的情况。

2.3 同位语从句的后移

除了主语后移和定语后移较常见外，同位语后移也是比较常见的现象。同位语从句的经典位置是在先行词之后，但在医学英语写作中，同位语特别复杂而述谓部分只有谓语动词而无宾语时，同位语从句有时会被放置到谓语之后，造成先行词与同位语从句隔离的情况。例如：

例 16：After an X ray examination，the question arose whether this patient should undergo an operation immediately.

做完 X 光检查后，病人的问题在于是否要立即动手术。

例 17：Evidence is emerging that plant fibers have profound influences on human nutrition because they alter the absorption and metabolism of many nutrients.

有迹象表明，植物纤维对人类的营养吸收颇有影响，因为它们能使很多营养物质的吸收与代谢发生变化。

后移对句子结构以及句子的含义产生了很大的影响，写作者对后移的种种现象和方法的掌握程度直接影响对英语语言的理解和运用。因此，我们在医学英语写作中要重视这一现象，要讲地道的英语，写规范的句子，以寻求对意义的正确理解与表达。

第三节 错例分析

例 1：Whether the level of clinical risk of breast cancer recurrence adds prognostic information to the recurrence score is not known.

尚不清楚乳腺癌复发的临床风险水平是否会增加复发评分的预后信息。

分析：例句的主语从句虽然充分介绍了句子信息，但与短小的谓语部分相比显得极不平衡，可以使用形式主语 there 或 it，后移主语从句。本句选择 there 作主语，可修改如下：

改为：There is no conclusion on whether the level of clinical risk of breast cancer recurrence adds prognostic information to the recurrence score.

例 2：To construct protoplasm in the lab has been attempted many times.
已多次尝试在实验室里构造原生质。

分析：本句主语为不定式短语 to construct protoplasm in the lab，可将主语后移，句首用 it 作形式主语，从而使句子的结构变得匀称，并且使后移的主语得到了强调。

改为：It has been attempted many times to construct protoplasm in the lab.

例 3：Special care must be taken of the patients who have just been operated on with heart disease.
对刚动过手术的患有心脏病的病人必须给予特别照顾。

分析：本句中心词 patients 既有短语 with heart disease，又有从句 who have just been operated on 作定语修饰，此时应将短语前置，从句置后，保持句子的紧凑感。

改为：Special care must be taken of the patients with heart disease who have just been operated on.

例 4：A five-year follow up study on a case of chronic myeloid leukemia diagnosed in 1971 in a man of 19 years old is reported.
1971 年，一位 19 岁青年被诊断为患有慢性粒细胞白血病，本文报道了对此病例的 5 年随访研究。

分析：介词短语 on a case of chronic myeloid leukemia 在句中作定语，修饰中心词 study，谓语动词 is reported 应紧跟主语之后，否则本句主语太长而谓语太短，不符合英语表达习惯。

改为：A five-year follow up study is reported on a case of chronic myeloid leukemia diagnosed in 1971 in a man of 19 years old.

例 5：Few data to support the efficacy of hepatocellular carcinoma surveillance in these patients is available.
很少有数据支持对这些患者进行肝细胞癌监测的有效性。

分析：本句主语后面带有不定式短语作定语，并无问题，但看完全句，比照了主语谓语，我们会发现，主语和谓语相距太远，被长定语隔离，不利于读者对句子的理解。将 to support the efficacy ... 后移，谓语动词 is available 紧跟主语之后，句子将更好理解。

改为：Few data is available to support the efficacy of hepatocellular carcinoma surveillance in these patients.

例 6：Tumours that display both hepatocytic and cholangiocytic differentiation represent a distinct entity, termed combined hepatocellular carcinoma cholangiocarcinoma.

同时显示肝细胞和胆管细胞分化的肿瘤是一种不同的肿瘤，称为合并肝细胞癌胆管癌。

分析：本句宾语 a distinct entity 有个过去分词 termed ... 作后置定语，然而 termed 后面紧跟的疾病名称又恰恰包含了过去分词 combined，这就出现了两个过去分词相邻，容易造成歧义，应想办法通过词序调整，使这个后移的定语发生变化，去除歧义。改动较小的方法是将后置定语 termed 改成其他词，例如 known as；或者也可以将句子做进一步分析，对语序做较大调整，使得整个句子清晰易解。

改为：Tumours that were termed combined hepatocellular carcinoma cholangio-carcinoma display both hepatocytic and cholangiocytic differentiation and represent a distinct entity.

例 7：A 48-year-old man having long-standing type 2 diabetes mellitus and chronic kidney disease presented with a 3-month history of numbness, tingling, and faint violaceous discoloration at the tips of multiple fingers and toes.

48 岁男性，长期患有 2 型糖尿病和慢性肾脏疾病，多个手指和脚趾有麻木和刺痛感达 3 个月之久，并且颜色呈现为紫色。

分析：医学论文中的语句在描述患者病症和临床表现时常常依赖某些介词使限定成分后移，例如介词 of 和 with。本句主语中心词 man 后面用现在分词 having ... 作后置定语，可改为 with 引出病症；例句的另一处介词误用也出现在后置定语的位置，discoloration 前面已经有两个形容词定语，那么限定该词的"手指、脚趾"就不便再叠加使用，而应当后移，但作者选择介词 at 帮助后移 the tips ... 却不妥当，因为 at the tips 的意思是"以指尖捏住"，引申为唾手可得，比如 The contact lens is placed at the tip of a finger（将隐形眼镜置于指尖），而例句想表达的是指/趾头本身的尖端部位发生变色，因此后置定语应选择介词 of 或者 in 引导。

改为：A 48-year-old man with long-standing type 2 diabetes mellitus and chronic kidney disease presented with a 3-month history of numbness, tingling, and faint violaceous discoloration of the tips of multiple fingers and toes.

第四节 练习巩固

1. 阅读下列句子,思考定语成分的位置,调整语序对后移进行修改。

(1) Despite the limitations of a small sample size, our data support the hypothesis based on lower rates of hospitalization and supplemental oxygen requirements that ADT may limit severe complications from acute pneumonia.

_____

(2) That new CAR-T cells will be developed to treat previously incurable human diseases is anticipated.

_____

(3) Specific recommendations in the criteria for dementia or AD with respect to what constitutes specific domains are not available.

_____

2. 阅读下列句子,填入适当的介词完成定语成分后移。

(1) There is echocardiographic evidence _____ structural remodeling that is most likely associated _____ chronic hypertension and alcohol use, but no clinical signs of heart failure are present.

(2) PCI can lead to worse clinical outcomes _____ patients _____ complex artery lesions.

(3) In this trial, we examined the risk-adjusted survival _____ 6 months after transplantation with a donor heart that had been reanimated and assessed _____ the use of extracorporeal nonischemic perfusion _____ circulatory death.

3. 翻译下列句子,注意定语后移。

(1) 本研究突出了基于已知的 H1N5 细胞进入和复制生物学的潜在治疗策略。

_____

(2) 需要新的方法以确认疾病的存在并提供有关疾病的严重程度和形态特征的信息。

_____

(3) 多数继续化疗的糖尿病患者显示肿瘤消退。

_____

第六章　关系从句

第一节　引言

1.1　定义

　　从属结构(subordination)是现代英语最重要的特点之一,同时也是中国英语学习者在学习与使用英语过程中的难点。关系从句(relative clause)又称定语从句,是提供关于先行词(名词、名词短语或代词)的描述性信息的从属分句。关系从句由关系词(关系代词或关系副词)引导。

　　关系从句作为从属结构的表现形式之一,在正式文体,尤其是在学术科研论文写作中得以广泛使用。学会正确使用关系从句,对提升学术英语写作的表达效果极为必要。

1.2　先行词

　　先行词(antecedent)指的是被关系从句修饰的对象,通常是发挥名词功能的语法单位,常见的先行词有名词、名词短语以及代词等。这正符合了"形容词修饰名词"这一基本的词性搭配规律。需要注意的是,先行词在主句中充当一定的语法成分。之所以被称为"先行词",是因为修饰它的关系从句总是放在它之后,先行词总是出现在关系从句之前。

　　例 1:For unvaccinated <u>individuals</u> who have not been previously infected with the flu, e. g. , the pediatric population, a bivalent vaccine approach may be particularly suitable.

　　对于以前未感染过流感并且未接种疫苗的个体,例如儿童群体,二价疫苗方法可能特别适合。

　　本句中,关系代词 who 引导的定语从句修饰先行词 individuals。

　　例 2:Myositis disease activity was assessed according to a core set of six <u>measures</u> that were designed for use in the evaluation of myositis.

依据专门设计用来评估肌炎的六种核心指标对肌炎疾病活动进行评估。

本句中,关系从句由 that 引导,修饰先行词 measures。

1.3 关系词

引导关系从句的关系词分为关系代词和关系副词,关系词被用来引导关系从句,代替关系从句所修饰的先行词,在关系从句中充当某个成分,如主语、宾语、定语等。

常见的关系词有关系代词(relative pronouns):that、which、who、whom;关系限定词(relative determiner):whose;关系副词(relative adverbs):where、when、why 等。

关系代词一般在从句中作主语、宾语、定语等。关系代词在从句中作主语时,从句谓语动词的人称和数要和先行词保持一致。此外,需要注意:关系副词有其常见的变体:why=for which;where=in/at/on/... which;when=during/on/in/... which。

例 3:As different mutations occur constantly, the term "variant" has been used to denote viral strains that carry a series of emerging amino acid mutations.

由于不断发生不同的突变,"变体"一词被用来表示携带一系列新出现的氨基酸突变的病毒株。

本句中,关系词 that 在关系从句作主语,谓语动词 carry 需要与先行词 strains 保持数的一致性。

例 4:However, the percentage of admissions that involved patients who were non-Hispanic was higher in the statewide group than in the weighted random sample.

然而,在全州范围内,涉及非西班牙裔患者的入院比例高于加权随机样本。

本句中存在两个关系从句结构,先行词分别指物和人,关系代词分别使用了 that 和 who。

此外,需要注意的是,有些情况只能使用关系代词 that,如:

(1) 先行词是不定代词 everything、anything、nothing、few、all、none、little、some 等;

(2) 先行词被序数词或 the last 修饰;

(3) 先行词被形容词最高级修饰;

(4) 先行词被 every、each、few、all、no、some、any、little、much 等修饰;

(5) 先行词被 the only、the very、the same 等修饰;

(6) 当先行词前面有 who、which 等疑问代词时;

(7) 当先行词既有人,也有物体时。

1.4 类别

关系从句由关系词(关系代词或关系副词)引导,其提供的信息对主句的完整性来说可能是必需的,也可能只是附加说明性的,由此可以把关系从句分为两大类:限定性关系从句（restrictive relative clause/defining relative clause）和非限定性关系从句（non-restrictive relative clause/non-defining relative clause）。如果关系从句起到限定说明、约束先行词的作用，我们称这类关系从句为限定性关系从句。限定性关系从句对主句中的先行词限定制约，使得先行词的意思更加明确具体，是句中不可或缺的部分。如果关系从句跟先行词的关系不是那么密切，只是为先行词提供一些补充的信息，起到附加说明的作用，我们把这类关系从句称为非限定性关系从句，即使去掉，也不影响主句意思的完整性。在非限定性关系从句中，一般需要用逗号把主句和从句分开，如果非限定性关系从句处在整个句子中间，前后都需要用逗号隔开。值得注意的是，非限定性关系从句的关系词不能使用 that。

1.5　英汉关系句式构建对比

对中国的英语学习者来说，使用英语写作之前有必要了解英汉两种语言之间最基本的不同。就汉语和英语而言，也许在语言学上最重要的区别就是形合和意合的对比。尽管汉语和英语都有形合句和意合句，但英语侧重形合，汉语更侧重意合。

汉语中没有关系从句，略于形式，偏重意会。汉语中的主从关系常常借助语序、上下文和副词等手段来表达，较少用连接词，汉语的定语一般在名词的前面，通常不使用关系从句。英语的修饰语在许多情况下可以通过形态变化或借助表示从属关系的关系代词和关系副词来表达，英语表达几乎离不开这些关系代词和关系副词。英语句子中的定语位置比较灵活，可以前置，也可以后置，后置的从句可以很长。英语句子呈现句首封闭、句尾开放的特征。

1.6　关系从句在医学学术英语写作中的使用

语言的意义单位是句子，在考虑语言结构时需要凸显句法的重要性。语言使用的目的在于传递信息，如何通过精心构撰的语言文字准确地传递丰富的信息是每一位语言使用者需要思考的问题。繁复的主从复合句是英语的特点之一，对医学英语写作尤其如此。医学学术语篇旨在对医学领域的研究与发展进行陈述，其语言表达必须客观准确，具有较强的逻辑性和严谨的结构。就关系从句而言，正确使用关系词有助于使句与句之间脉络清晰，条理自然，帮助读者准确理解论文的思路。

第二节　举例说明

2.1　限定性关系从句

例 1：This digital infrastructure would facilitate the most effective use of new vaccines and injectable therapies that could transform the prevention agenda and improve pandemic preparedness.

这一数字基础设施将有助于最有效地使用新疫苗和注射疗法,从而改变预防议程并改善疫情准备。

例 2：Vaccination strategies that can induce more potent, more durable, and broader immune responses are important to enhance protection.

能够诱导更有效、更持久和更广泛的免疫反应的疫苗接种策略对加强保护非常重要。

例 3：The process of cancer immunosurveillance is a mechanism of tumor suppression that can protect the host from cancer development throughout its lifetime.

癌症免疫监测的过程是一种肿瘤抑制机制,可以保护宿主在其整个生命周期中免受癌症侵扰。

从以上例句可以看出,有了关系从句的限定与约束,先行词的意思变得更加具体,如果去掉限定性关系从句,主句的含义往往会变得不完整或不明确。

2.2 非限定性关系从句

例 4：These hospitals all had the same malpractice insurance carrier, which provided support for this study as a component of its mission.

这些医院都有相同的医疗事故保险公司,作为其使命的一部分,该公司为这项研究提供支持。

例 5：However, the study was not designed to evaluate vaccine effectiveness, and the follow-up time of infection after the booster is limited, which precludes conclusions about protection.

然而,该研究的目的不是评估疫苗的有效性,而且接种加强针感染后的随访时间有限,排除了关于保护的结论。

例 6：Identification of interventions, both during critical care and after critical care, which improve recovery from critical illness, has been recognized as a priority by patients and their caregivers.

确定危重症患者在重症监护期间和重症监护后的干预措施,以促进其康复,已被患者及其护理人员视为优先事项。

从以上例句可以看出,非限定性关系从句用逗号与主句分开,起附加说明作用,如果去掉,不影响主句含义的完整性。

第三节 错例分析

例 1：The overall incidences of adverse events that was considered by the investigator to be related to vaccination study were 5.7% and 5.8% in the respective groups.

研究人员认为与疫苗接种研究相关的不良事件的总发生率分别为 5.7% 和 5.8%。

分析：写好关系从句非常重要的一点就是要确定需要限定、修饰的先行词，然后依据先行词来确定关系从句中的关系词，以及从句中主谓一致的问题，本句中先行词为"events"，所以从句中的"was"应该改为"were"。

改为：The overall incidences of adverse events that were considered by the investigator to be related to vaccination study were 5.7% and 5.8% in the respective groups.

例 2：The first key step when doing a diagnostic assessment is to establish a trusting relationship with the young person which can require time and effort——especially if the young person has been reluctant to seek help.

进行诊断评估的第一个关键步骤是与年轻人建立信任关系，这可能需要时间和精力，尤其是在年轻人不愿寻求帮助的情况下。

分析：结合前文对限定性关系从句与非限定性关系从句的分析可以看出，在关系代词"which"前需要加一个逗号，将从句改为非限定关系从句，此时句子中的先行词是句子"The first key step when doing a diagnostic assessment is to establish a trusting relationship with the young person"，which 指代这个句子。

改为：The first key step when doing a diagnostic assessment is to establish a trusting relationship with the young person, which can require time and effort——especially if the young person has been reluctant to seek help.

例 3：Every patient with valvular or congenital heart disease which develops an obscure fever which persists for more than a few days should be suspected.

任何瓣膜性或先天性心脏病患者，如出现原因不明的发热，并持续多天，即应加以怀疑。

分析：该句中修饰成分包括一个介词短语 with valvular or congenital heart disease 与两个定语从句，结构相对复杂。根据句子内容与结构可以看出，第一个关系从句修饰的先行词应为 every patient，所以应当把第一个 which 改为 who。

改为：Every patient with valvular or congenital heart disease who develops an obscure fever which persists for more than a few days should be suspected.

例 4：The diseases which primary carcinoma of the liver must be differentiated are metastatic tumour, cirrhosis and abscess of the liver.

必须与原发性肝癌鉴别的疾病是转移性肿瘤、肝硬化和肝脓肿。

分析：关系从句的谓语动词为含有介词的动词短语，且先行词在从句中作介词的宾语时，该介词可以移到关系代词之前，构成"介词＋which/whom"引导的关系从句句式。结合从句中的 differentiate 一词的用法，此句应在关系代词 which 前加上 from。需要注意的是，在一些含有介词的短语动词中，由于动词与介词的关系比较紧密（如：listen to、take care of、get rid of、look forward to 等），一般不能将介词与动词分开，故而也不能将介词提到关系代词之前。

改为：The diseases from which primary carcinoma of the liver must be differentiated are metastatic tumour, cirrhosis and abscess of the liver.

第四节　练习巩固

1. 划出下列句子中的关系从句。

（1）One study showed a measured incidence that was almost 20 times as high as the incidence identified through voluntary reporting.

（2）The immune system provides sophisticated defense mechanisms that most often eliminate or contain the appearance of tumor cells in healthy tissue, and prevent the development of life-threatening cancers.

（3）Commercial tools which can identify some types of harm in hospitalized patients, including adverse drug events and health care-associated infections, are already available and widely used.

（4）Cognitive behavioral therapy that includes behavior activation, caregiver involvement, and challenging cognitive distortions is more effective than cognitive behavioral therapy that exclusively focuses on cognitive distortions.

（5）A noninvasive technology that quantitatively measures the extent of brain cholesterol metabolism could broadly affect disease diagnosis and treatment options using targeted therapies.

2. 请把下面的中文句子翻译成英文，注意务必使用关系从句。

（1）在我们的研究中，我们确定了 10 个导致不良事件的诊断错误。

（2）主要发现包括，每100例入院患者中有3.7起不良事件，其中28%被认为是由疏忽造成的。

_____

（3）这种方法依赖于对大量病毒序列的分析，目前只有少数病原体可以公开获得这些序列。

_____

（4）识别肿瘤抗原的 T 细胞对增强抗肿瘤免疫反应至关重要。

_____

3. 请把下面的句子翻译成中文，注意关系从句的结构。

（1）The presence of depressive symptoms that do not meet full diagnostic criteria for major depressive disorder is known as subthreshold depression, which has negative effects on quality of life and is a risk indicator of a later depressive disorder.

_____

（2）Ten percent of the adverse events that had been identified were randomly selected to be judged by a second physician.

_____

（3）We placed mice at thermoneutrality（30℃），which is defined as the temperature at which mice expend minimal energy on maintaining body temperature.

_____

（4）Natural killer（NK）cells are described as "innate lymphocytes that can kill virally infected or tumorigenic cells without prior sensitization."

_____

（5）These findings agree with previous findings，which demonstrated a reduction in the number of transmission clusters and the risk of transmission.

_____

第七章　非谓语动词

第一节　引言

1.1　定义

非谓语动词,又叫非限定动词(non-finite forms of the verb),是指在句子中不是谓语的动词,主要包括动词不定式(to do)、现在分词(doing)和过去分词(done)、动名词(doing)。

非谓语动词也是动词的一种,除了不能独立作谓语外,可以承担句子的其他成分,如主语、宾语、状语等。非谓语动词可以强化句子的语法结构,增加句子的丰富度和表达力。通过使用非谓语动词,可以更清楚地表达出动作发生的方式、原因、目的或时间。

1.2　形式

非谓语动词形式上相对比较稳定,主要分为以下几种:

不定式是动词的基本形式,常常由 to 加上动词原形构成。在句子中可以作为主语、宾语、表语、定语、补语等。

分词分为现在分词和过去分词两种形式,现在分词是动词的-ing 形式,过去分词主要是动词的-ed 形式,部分过去分词的形式则根据动词的不同规则变化。分词可以作为形容词使用,修饰名词或代词。

动名词是动词加上-ing 形式的现在分词。在句子中可以作为主语、宾语、表语、定语、补语等。

常见的语态和形式如下表:

	语态	一般式	完成式	进行式
动词不定式	主动	to do	to have done	to be doing
	被动	to be done	to have been done	

	语态	一般式	完成式	进行式
现在分词	主动	doing	having done	
	被动	being done	having been done	
过去分词	被动	done		
动名词	主动	doing		

在医学英语中,非谓语动词的使用非常常见。例如:

- After **finishing**(动名词) medical school, she started her residency.
- He decided **to specialize**(不定式) in cardiology.
- The injured patient, **lying**(现在分词) on the hospital bed, was in great pain.
- Prenatal vitamins are important for the health of the **developing**(现在分词作定语) fetus.
- With a **broken**(过去分词作定语) leg, she couldn't walk properly.

1.3 作用

非谓语动词在句子中可以起到补充信息、补充说明、修饰限定等作用,丰富句子结构,拓展句子表达能力。英语书面表达中出现过多的简单句会让人觉得单调乏味,句子与句子之间的关系显得松散;而文章中过多地出现复合句又显得累赘,读起来费劲。有效地使用词句间的连接成分,使全文结构紧凑从而达到预期的写作目的,恰当地应用非谓语动词对简单句和复合句进行转换,不仅可使句型多样,而且可使句子结构紧凑,言简意明。因此,非谓语动词在书面表达中的重要性不言而喻。

在医学英语论文中,非谓语动词常用于描述实验方法、研究结果以及分析和讨论等方面。在写作医学英语论文时,正确使用非谓语动词可以更准确地传达信息,让语言更加简洁且具有条理性,有助于表达科学事实和推理。

第二节 举例说明

2.1 动词不定式

例 1:Further research is needed **to understand** the similarities and differences in the clinical and biological characteristics of patients with ARDS (Acute Respiratory Distress Syndrome) and acute hypoxaemic respiratory failure.

还需要进一步的研究,来了解 ARDS(急性呼吸窘迫综合征)患者和急性低氧性呼吸衰竭患者,在临床和生物学特征上的相似性和差异性。

例 2：The results seem **to have confirmed** the effectiveness of the new treatment method for chronic pain.

结果似乎已经证实了这种新治疗方法对慢性疼痛的有效性。

例 3：The intervention was designed **to be facilitating** better communication between healthcare providers and patients.

该干预措施旨在促进医疗工作者与患者之间更好地沟通。

例 4：Symptoms of depression have been found **to be associated with** eating disorders and functional somatic symptoms.

研究发现，抑郁症的症状和进食障碍以及功能性躯体症状有关。

例 5：The change in the disease progression was found **to have been significantly correlated** with the levels of the inflammatory biomarker.

研究发现，疾病进展的变化与炎症生物标志物的水平存在显著相关性。

2.2　现在分词

例 6：**Having conducted** thorough research and careful analysis，the authors concluded that the new treatment method was effective in reducing symptoms of depression.

经过深入研究和仔细分析，作者得出结论：新的治疗方法在减轻抑郁症症状方面是有效的。

例 7：**Being done** prospectively，this study will follow a cohort of patients over a period of five years to assess the long-term outcomes of a new treatment approach.

本研究将对一组患者进行为期五年的随访，以评估一种新治疗方法的长期效果，研究具有前瞻性。

例 8：**Having been administered** the experimental drug，the rats exhibited improved cognitive function.

在服用了实验药物后，大鼠的认知功能有所改善。

2.3　过去分词

例 9：**Elevated** serum levels of insulin-like growth factor-1 （IGF-1） in postmenopausal women have been associated with an **increased** risk of breast cancer.

绝经后妇女血清中胰岛素样生长因子-1(IGF-1)水平增高与乳腺癌风险增加有关。

例 10：The study utilized a **randomized**，double-blind，placebo-**controlled** design，aiming to assess the efficacy of the investigational drug in reducing symptoms of post-traumatic stress disorder.

该研究采用了随机、双盲、安慰剂对照的设计，旨在评估研究药物在减轻创伤后应激障碍症状方面的疗效。

2.4 动名词

例 11：The reaction mixture was incubated overnight at 4 ℃ to allow for optimal **binding** between the antibody and target antigen.

反应混合物在 4 ℃下孵育过夜，以便于抗体与靶抗原之间的最佳结合。

例 12：The study aimed at **investigating** the effects of **implementing** a standardized patient education program on **enhancing** self-care management among older adults living with diabetes.

这项研究旨在调查标准化病人教育项目的实施对提高老年糖尿病患者自我管理能力的影响。

第三节　错例分析

例 1：Despite experienced some complications during surgery, the patient showed significant improvement in their overall health and wellbeing post-operation.

尽管手术中出现了一些并发症，但患者在手术后的整体健康和福祉方面有了明显的改善。

分析：本句话的主句是 the patient showed significant improvement ... ，showed 是谓语动词，其他部分出现动词都只能使用非谓语动词形式，despite 后边只能接名词或动名词组成介词短语，不能使用动词过去式 experienced，应将 experienced 改为 experiencing。

改为：Despite experiencing some complications during surgery, the patient showed significant improvement in their overall health and wellbeing post-operation.

例 2：To improve the understanding of the pathological mechanisms underlie the disease, the study employed various molecular and cellular techniques to investigate the expression and function of key proteins in affected tissues.

为了提高对疾病病理机制的理解，该研究采用了各种分子和细胞技术来研究受影响组织中关键蛋白质的表达和功能。

分析：To improve the understanding of the pathological mechanisms underlie the disease 这里的 underlie 不是谓语动词，不可以使用动词原形，应改为现在分词 underlying 或者定语从句结构 that underlie，作为后置定语或者定语从句修饰 pathological mechanisms。

改为：To improve the understanding of the pathological mechanisms underlying /

that underlie the disease, the study employed various molecular and cellular techniques to investigate the expression and function of key proteins in affected tissues.

例 3：Chronic obstructive pulmonary disease is characterized by persistent airway inflammation, causing narrow of the airways, leading to reduced airflow and impaired gas exchange.

慢性阻塞性肺病的特征是持续的气道炎症，导致气道狭窄，进而导致气流减少和气体交换受损。

分析：Causing narrow of the airways 中 cause 后边只跟名词或者动名词，表示造成或导致的症状，narrow 本身是动词或形容词，需要改成动名词形式 narrowing。

改为：Chronic obstructive pulmonary disease is characterized by persistent airway inflammation, causing narrowing of the airways, leading to reduced airflow and impaired gas exchange.

第四节　练习巩固

1. 划出下列句子中的非谓语动词成分。

（1）In this cross-sectional analysis, we examined the association between physical activity levels and markers of cardiovascular disease risk, such as elevated blood pressure and cholesterol levels.

（2）The cohort was comprised of healthy individuals without a history of cardiovascular disease, with ages ranging from 18 to 65 years old.

（3）Vascular endothelial growth factor plays a crucial role in angiogenesis, the process of forming new blood vessels from pre-existing ones, which is essential in tissue repair and wound healing.

（4）Despite the limitations of this study, the results obtained from the samples collected from the populations under investigation strongly advise for a more comprehensive evaluation of the potential benefits of the therapy being tested.

（5）The participants of the clinical trial were selected based on specific criteria, having been diagnosed with the condition under investigation.

2. 请根据上下文用括号中词语的正确形式补充完成下列句子。

（1）The study results revealed that individuals with a history of smoking had a higher risk of ＿＿＿＿＿＿（develop）lung cancer, as confirmed by various epidemiological studies.

(2) The data analysis showed a statistically significant difference in the average recovery time between patients _____ (treat) with the new therapy and those receiving the standard treatment.

(3) _____ (determine) the efficacy of the novel therapeutic intervention, the study aimed _____ (recruit) a large and diverse sample of patients with varying disease severity and demographic characteristics.

(4) To investigate the role of epigenetic modifications in the pathogenesis of autoimmune diseases, genome-wide DNA methylation and histone modification profiles were generated from blood samples _____ (obtain) from both patients and healthy controls.

(5) The findings suggest that _____ (engage) patients in shared decision-making processes regarding treatment options can improve treatment adherence and patient outcomes.

3. 请把下面的中文句子翻译成英文，注意适当使用非谓语动词。

(1) 一些研究已经显示,结果很有希望。目前研究人员正在进行更多的调查。

_____

(2) 这项研究旨在探究新药物的潜在副作用。

_____

(3) 这项研究的目的是确定一种新疗法在减轻症状方面的有效性。

_____

(4) 研究人员分析了从研究参与者那里收集到的数据。

_____

(5) 我们进行了全面的文献回顾,来确定在过去五年内已经发表的相关研究。

_____

第八章 标点符号

第一节 引言

1.1 标点符号对学术论文的重要性

一篇学术论文质量的高低无疑取决于它的学术水平,即作者的学术功底和创新能力,但是语言文字表达也是重要依据之一,而规范使用标点符号则体现了学术论文的基本功。所以,英文学术论文撰写者,除了要保证文章语法正确、用词精准、流畅地道等外,同样不可忽视英文标点符号的使用。美国的标准化考试 SAT 和 ACT 也指明要考标点符号的用法,标点符号对于英文写作的重要性可见一斑。

1.2 标点符号对期刊质量的重要性

国内期刊对中文标点符号的使用制定了详细权威的标准规范,然而对英文标点符号的用法尚无统一、官方的标准可遵循,导致国内学术期刊里英文标点符号使用错误频现,这实际上也制约着国内学术期刊的发展。一篇标点使用不规范的论文也常常令审稿专家和期刊编辑感到棘手,无法修改,从而增加了论文被拒的风险。

尽管国际上关于英文标点符号尚无统一标准,美国和英国的标点符号在使用习惯上也有不同,但对于常用的标点符号,还是存在一定的共识。由于篇幅有限,本章不打算全面介绍英文标点符号的使用规则,而是结合中英文标点的差异,通过对学术论文撰写和期刊编辑中常见的错误进行分析和探讨,简要介绍标点符号使用的注意事项,旨在引起学术论文作者对此问题的重视。

第二节　举例说明

2.1　并列成分中逗号的使用

（1）通常不用逗号连接只有两个并列的成分，但当名词前的定语是两个并列的形容词时，可用逗号连接，不加连词。但在累积形容词之间不能使用逗号。

例 1：The American Academy of Pediatrics Guidance encourages caregivers to create safe, nurturing environments by avoiding spanking and establishing routines.

《美国儿科学会指南》鼓励看护人通过避免责打和建立常规生活来创造安全的、有益的环境。

例 2：It is still far from the development of a completely protective practical successful AIDS vaccine.

还远未开发出一种完全具有保护性且实际成功的艾滋病疫苗。

注意，例 2 名词 AIDS vaccine 前面是两个累积形容词，之间无需用逗号连接。

（2）有时为了避免误解，在两个并列成分中间除了使用连词，还可以加逗号。

例 3：A few studies have examined the interaction of exposures to adverse childhood experiences and positive childhood experiences, and the differential impacts on anxiety, depression, and comorbid anxiety-depression.

一些研究调查了暴露于不良童年经历和积极童年经历之间的相互作用，以及对焦虑、抑郁和共病焦虑—抑郁的不同影响。

注意，例 3 标示处的逗号提示 impacts 连接的对象不是较近的 experiences，而是较远的 interaction。

2.2　并列复合句中标点符号的使用

（1）两个独立的句子不能单用逗号连接，还需要用连词，如 and、but、or、so、yet、while、whereas 等。

例 4：The more recent study indicated that in 2006 the worldwide total number of patients with Alzheimer's disease was 26.6 million, and by 2050 the number will quadruple.

最近的一项研究表明，2006 年全球阿尔茨海默病患者总数为 2660 万，而到 2050 年这一数字将增加四倍。

例 5：Alzheimer's disease is an inevitable consequence of aging, <u>whereas</u> a convergence to or a decline at certain age may suggest that very old people may have reduced vulnerability, owing perhaps to genetic or environmental factors.

阿尔茨海默病是衰老造成的，<u>而</u>在一定年龄时的趋同或下降可能表明，高龄老人可能已经降低了脆弱性，这可能受遗传或环境影响。

（2）句中有承接词时，需要注意标点符号的应用

常见的承接词有承接并列关系的，如 also、then、moreover、furthermore、in addition、besides；承接因果关系的，如 thus、therefore、hence、consequently、as a result；承接转折关系的，如 however、nevertheless。承接词是副词，不能单独用来构成并列复合句，也不可用逗号加承接词来构成复合句。有承接词时可采用以下三种连接方式：用分号连接；写成独立的句子，句首用大写；如用逗号，则需另加连词 and 或 but 等。以下例句有两种或多种连接方式：

例 6：（1）The authors did not consider types of ACEs and PCEs in their adjusted models; <u>therefore</u>, future research should comprehensively examine the interacting effect of each type of ACE and PCE on the outcome of internalizing behavior.

（2）The authors did not consider types of ACEs and PCEs in their adjusted models. <u>Therefore</u>, future research should comprehensively examine the interacting effect of each type of ACE and PCE on the outcome of internalizing behavior.

（3）The authors did not consider types of ACEs and PCEs in their adjusted models, <u>and therefore</u>, future research should comprehensively examine the interacting effect of each type of ACE and PCE on the outcome of internalizing behavior.

作者在他们调整后的模型中没有考虑 ACEs 和 PCEs 类型。<u>因此</u>，未来研究应全面研究各类型的 ACE 和 PCE 对内化行为结果的交互作用。

例 7：（1）Evidence appears to be stronger for aerobic exercise; <u>however</u>, there is also some supportive evidence for resistance training and other forms of exercise.

（2）Evidence appears to be stronger for aerobic exercise. <u>However</u>, there is also some supportive evidence for resistance training and other forms of exercise.

关于有氧运动的证据似乎更有力。<u>然而</u>，也有一些支持阻力训练和其他形式运动的证据。

注意，however 后不可接转折连词 but，因此例 7 如用 however 承接，则只有两种连接方式。

2.3　句首有状语时逗号的使用

（1）位于句首的状语或状语从句，可用逗号与主句隔开。

例 8：<u>Additionally,</u> by asking participants to rate their experience in the past, it is possible that responses were affected by recall bias and fluctuations over time.

此外，通过要求参与者评价他们过去的经历，他们的评价可能受到回忆偏差和随时间推移变化的影响。

例 9：<u>Because occurrence of AD is strongly associated with increasing age,</u> it is anticipated that this dementing disorder will pose huge challenges to public health and elderly care systems in all countries across the world.

由于 AD 的发生与年龄的增长密切相关，预计这种痴呆障碍将对世界上各国的公共卫生和老年人护理系统构成巨大挑战。

（2）在倒装句中，位于句首的状语或状语从句均不可用逗号与主句隔开。

例 10：Only in two cases was breast cancer discovered, grade 1 in one and grade 3 in the other.

只发现两例乳腺癌，一例 1 级，另一例 3 级。

注意，in two cases 后不可加逗号。

例 11：Not until the food has entered the blood and been used by the tissue cells can the body be said to have accepted it.

食物在未进入血液并未被组织细胞利用之前，还不能说食物已被机体所接受。

注意，在 the tissue cells 后不可用逗号。

2.4　冒号的使用

（1）冒号可用来引出一系列并列成分或句子，冒号前可以是完整的句子，也可以是不完整的句子。

例 12：Participants were compensated according to their level of compliance with the EMA procedures：they were paid ＄250 for completion of 75％—100％ of the prompted diaries, ＄170 for 50％—74％, ＄100 for 25％—49％, and ＄50 for 0％—25％.

参与者根据他们遵守 EMA 程序的程度获得补偿：他们完成 75％—100％的提示日志得到 250 美元，完成 50％—74％获得 170 美元，完成 25％—49％获得 100 美元，完成 0％—25％获得 50 美元。

例 13：Mean daily intakes on the low fiber diets were：zinc, 11.2 mg；copper, 1.6 mg；phosphorus, 1.542 g.

低纤维饮食的平均日摄入量为：锌，11.2 毫克；铜，1.6 毫克；磷，1.542 克。

（2）冒号后的各并列成分之前还可以加数字、英语字母以及罗马字母等表示顺序。

例 14：The 2-year multidomain interventions include four main components：(i) nutritional guidance；(ii) physical activity；(iii) cognitive training and social activity；and (iv) intensive monitoring and management of metabolic and vascular risk factors.

为期两年的多领域干预措施包括四个主要组成部分：（i）营养指导；（ii）体育活动；（iii）认知训练和社会活动；以及（iv）对代谢和血管危险因素的强化监测和管理。

注意，在加用表示顺序的标志后，可以不用冒号。

2.5 括号的使用

（1）医学论文中的括号常有两种作用：表示同位关系或者用来补充说明。

例 15：Current medications widely used for AD and dementia are cholinesterase inhibitors (donepezil，rivastigmine，and galantamine) and the N-methyl-D-aspartate-receptor antagonist (memantine).

目前广泛用于治疗阿尔茨海默病和痴呆症的药物有胆碱酯酶抑制剂（多奈哌齐、瑞瓦斯替明和加兰他明）和 N-甲基-D-天冬氨酸受体拮抗剂（美金刚）。

例 16：While the original study measured three types of ACEs (i. e.，abuse，neglect，household dysfunction)，more recent studies have expanded these categories.

最初的研究评价了三种类型 ACEs（即虐待、忽视、家庭功能障碍），但最近的研究扩大了这些类别。

（2）括号中还可包含多种语法结构，如介词短语、分词短语、从属句，甚至完整的句子，来补充说明括号前所表述的内容。

例 17：The *Lancet* Commission emphasized the importance of a lifelong approach to dementia risk reduction，from childhood (increasing access and duration of education) through to older age (keeping physically and cognitively active).

《柳叶刀》委员会强调了终身降低痴呆症风险的重要性，从儿童期（增加教育机会和教育持续时间）到老年（保持身体活动和认知活动）。

例 18：At each diary entry，participants were asked to respond to questions inquiring about the presence of NSSI urges(i. e.，In the past 4 h，have you had an urge to self-injure?) and behaviors (i. e.，Have you engaged in self-injurious behavior in the past 4 h?)

在每一篇日志中，参与者被要求回答有关自伤冲动存在的问题（即"在过去的 4 小时内你是否有自残的冲动?"）以及自残行为（即，"你在过去 4 小时内是否有过自残行为?"）。

第三节　错例分析

例 1：A literature search of electronic databases PsycINFO、CINAHL、MEDLINE, and Web of Science was performed from the earliest date available to March 2022.

检索电子数据库 PsycINFO、CINAHL、MEDLINE 和 Web of Science，检索的文献日期为从最早可查日期到 2022 年 3 月。

分析：此句中数据库名称之间不能用顿号连接，应将两处顿号改为逗号。英文中没有顿号，凡是顿号所表示的内容均用逗号表示。

改为：A literature search of electronic databases PsycINFO, CINAHL, MEDLINE, and Web of Science was performed from the earliest date available to March 2022.

例 2：A 18-year-old young man was admitted to hospital on July，23，2020，for evaluation of nasosinusitis.

一位 18 岁年轻男患者于 2020 年 7 月 23 日入院接受鼻窦炎检查。

分析：按月、日、年顺序表示的英文日期，年的前面需加逗号隔开，月和日之间不用逗号。按日、月、年顺序表达的日期则无需使用逗号。当只有年和月时，中间也无需用逗号隔开。因此，例 2 中 July 后的逗号需删除。

改为：A 18-year-old young man was admitted to hospital on July 23，2020，for evaluation of nasosinusitis.

例 3：It is imperative to maintain the highest possible population immunity level indefinitely, thus this plan may be the biggest flaw in the current strategy.

必须无限期地保持尽可能高的人口免疫水平，因此，该计划可能是当前战略中的最大缺陷。

分析：thus 作为承接词是副词，不能误当作连词来构成并列复合句。

改为：It is imperative to maintain the highest possible population immunity level indefinitely；thus，this plan … .

或者 It is imperative to maintain the highest possible population immunity level indefinitely. Thus, this plan … .

或者 It is imperative to maintain the highest possible population immunity level indefinitely, and thus, this plan … .

例 4：Ten weeks later, oral glucose tolerance test was performed in all groups, the change of rat body weight, fasting blood glucose and fasting serum insulin were routinely determined.

　　10 周后,各组均进行口服糖耐量试验,常规测定大鼠体重、空腹血糖、空腹血清胰岛素的变化情况。

　　分析:此句有两个独立的句子,中间用逗号连接不妥当,应将逗号改为分号,或者在逗号前加连词。

　　改为:... oral glucose tolerance test was performed in all groups. The change of ... .

　　或者... oral glucose tolerance test was performed in all groups, and the change of ... .

　　或者... oral glucose tolerance test was performed in all groups; the change of ... .

　　论文写作中要注意避免"逗号错"(comma fault),即用逗号代替句号、分号等。至于何时将逗号改为句号、分号,以及加何种连词,则视两个句子的逻辑关系而定。

第四节　练习巩固

1. 请给下列句子补上必要的标点符号。

(1) The median age of the patients was 65 years 108 patients were males.

(2) The advanced age hypertension diabetes atrial fibrillation and dyslipidemia are the most important risk factors for the recurrence of ischemic stroke.

(3) Importantly there is evidence that genetic risks of dementia may also be offset.

(4) Physical activity has additional indirect mechanisms on brain health through reducing vascular disease risk improving diabetes hypertension hypercholesterolaemia and obesity as well as reducing depression sleep disturbance and social isolation.

(5) Our patients were divided into three groups Group Ⅰ 44 patients without cells having convoluted neclei Group Ⅱ 30 patients with 10% or fewer convoluted nucleus cells CNC and Group Ⅲ 27 patients with more than 30% CNC.

2. 改正下列句子中使用错误的标点符号。

(1) Our data were collected from national adolescent new-risk behavior surveillance during May, 28, 2021 to December, 30, 2021.

(2) We found no evidence of invasive breast cancer, however, biopsy changes were detected in both groups.

(3) Alzheimer's disease—a progressive neurodegenerative disease, is characterized by

memory impairment and cognitive dysfunction.

（4）There are serious scientific questions that must be addressed，if we are to formulate future immunization policies tailored to different parts of the world.

（5）150 min of vigorous physical activity per week was found to be associated with a lower hazard ratio （0. 74；95％CI 0. 68 to 0. 81） of death over the 12 year follow up period.

医学英语写作语篇技能

第一章　医学研究论文的分类与组成

第一节　医学研究论文的分类

医学研究论文是研究者对某一个医学研究课题在理论、实证或临床治疗经验方面所取得的创新性研究成果或见解的科学记录和总结,是医学界同仁进行学术交流和研究的重要媒介。当前国际生物医学期刊绝大多数都以英文撰写,从体裁上来说,主要包括以下几种类型:

（1）论著（Original paper）

论著是作者将自己的科研成果或临床经验以严密的论证方法和合乎学术规范的语言编撰而成的研究性论文,属于一次性文献。论著包括实验研究、临床研究、临床报告等,是各种医学学术性期刊的核心部分。论著的正文通常由前言（Introduction）、材料和方法（Materials and Methods）、结果（Results）、讨论（Discussion）等几部分组成,国外取其首字母,简称为 IMRAD 格式,我们后面将重点描述。

（2）病例报告（Case report）

病例报告针对一例或数例典型病例进行描述和分析,介绍其发病表现、诊断标准和处理方法,总结其诊治经验,具备很强的临床实用价值,是医学期刊中常见的一个栏目。以往病例报告多是报道一些新发病例,如艾滋病、军团病都是通过病例报告的形式被医学界首次关注,如今针对已知疾病的特殊临床表现、影像学及检验学等诊断手段的新发现、疾病的特殊临床转归等也是病例报告的重点内容。

（3）综述（Review）

综述是就医学某一专题在一段时间内的文献数据、资料和主要观点进行分析总结、归纳提炼而成的文章,对作者和读者确定科研课题、把握研究方向均具有极其重要的参考价值。综述并不只是对文献资料的简单罗列,而是要能够做出全面、综合的分析,反映作者的观点与见解,做出有价值的评价。综述对作者的专业能力要求较高,有的期刊明确要求,只刊登编辑约稿,所以投稿之前请一定阅读投稿须知。

（4）评论（Commentary）

评论类文章是就某一观点或问题发表自己的见解,做出适当的评价。以《新英格兰医学杂志》（NEJM）为例,"Commentary"下属的文章有很多类型,如"Editorial"（编辑按)、"Perspective"(观点)、"Clinical Implications of Basic Research"(基础研究的临床意义)和"Letter to the Editor"(读者来信)等。每一种类型的文章也有相应的要求,如"perspective"类文章应以简短、通俗易懂的风格分析医学相关的较新话题,通常要求包含一个图表或表格,作者为一位或两位,不超过 1200 个单词,参考文献不宜超过 5 条;"Clinical Implications of Basic Research"类文章则要求作者讨论一篇别人撰写的临床前期论文,解释其研究结果并评论可能的临床应用,不得对自己的作品进行评论,最多含有一个图表,文章不超过 750 个单词,参考文献也不宜超过 5 条。

以上几种是比较常见的期刊文章类型,大家在投稿之前要清楚自己文章所属的类别,以便向相应栏目进行投稿。学术期刊网站上都有详细的投稿须知或告知作者(Guide for Authors),大家一定要仔细阅读,必要时可发邮件给编辑部进行咨询。

第二节 医学研究论文的组成

由于研究的目的、内容、要求和文章体裁的不同,医学研究论文的格式和写作方法也不完全一样,各自具有比较固定的格式。一般来说,医学研究论文组成部分如下表:

Section	Purpose
Title(标题)	What the paper is about
Authors(作者及单位)	Names and affiliations of authors
Abstract(摘要)	A stand-alone, short narrative of the paper
Key words(关键词)	Words other than those in title that best describe the paper
Introduction(前言)	Why this paper? The problem, what is not known, the objective of the study
Materials and Methods(材料与方法)	How was the study done?
Results(结果)	What did you find?
Discussion(讨论)	What does it mean? What next? Interpretation of results and future directions
Conclusion(结论)	Possible implications
Acknowledgments(致谢)	Who helped and how? What was the founding source?
References(参考文献)	Details of papers cited
Appendices(附录)	Supplementary materials

以上几项是医学论文的主要组成部分,此外有的医学论文还包括插图与说明(legends)、图表(figures)、表格(tables)、照片与说明(plates and explanations)等部分。

如前所述,论著类文章的正文通常由前言(Introduction)、材料和方法(Materials

and Methods)、结果(Results)、讨论(Discussion)等几部分组成,这是组成正文必不可少的几个部分,但根据各期刊编排和要求,排列顺序会有所不同,其中最为常见的即为 IMRAD 格式,其中每个字母分别代表 Introduction(前言)、Methods(研究方法)、Results(研究结果)、And(和)以及 Discussion(讨论)。如下图所示:

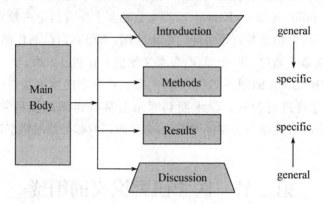

根据 IMRAD 格式,在撰写论著类文章每个部分时,应遵循以下规则:

Title(题目):

1. Describe contents clearly and precisely.

2. Provide key words for indexing.

3. Don't include wasted words such as "studies on", "an investigation of".

4. Don't include abbreviations and jargon.

Abstract(摘要):

1. State main objectives.

2. Describe methods.

3. Summarize the most important results.

4. State major conclusions and significance.

5. Find out maximum length.

Introduction(前言):

1. Describe the problem investigated.

2. Summarize relevant research to provide context, key terms, and concepts.

3. Move from general to specific: problem in research literature → your experiment.

4. Make clear the links between problem and solution, prior research and your experiment.

5. Be selective in choosing studies to cite and amount of detail to include.

Methods and Materials(方法和材料):

1. Briefly explain the general type of scientific procedure used.

2. Use subheadings to proceed.

3. Explain the steps taken in the experiments.

4. Provide enough detail for replication.

5. Use past tense to describe.

Results(结果)

1. Briefly describe experiment without detail of Methods section.

2. Report main results supported by selected data.

3. Order multiple results logically:from most to least important,from simple to complex.

4. Use past tense to describe.

5. Don't simply repeat table data;do select.

6. Don't interpret results.

Discussion(讨论)

1. Summarize the most important findings at the beginning.

2. Draw conclusions for each major result (eg:explain plausibly any agreements, contradictions, or exceptions).

3. Fit results into a broader context (eg: suggest theoretical implications or practical applications of results).

4. Move from specific to general:findings→literature, theory, practice.

5. Don't ignore or bury the major issue.

6. Don't overgeneralize.

7. Don't ignore deviations in data.

遵循以上论著类文章撰写所需要的原则,将会大大提高论文被期刊录用的概率。我们也将在后面的章节中,通过大量例文系统分析每一部分特定的写作要求,总结其语言特征和常用表达句型,意图帮助本书读者从内容和格式上提高论文写作质量。

第二章 标 题

第一节 标题的要求

1.1 标题的基本要求

标题是对论文内容的高度概括,既要简明扼要,又要引人注目。要写好论文的标题,应该达到以下几个基本要求:

(1) 主题明确

标题的含义应与论文的内容相吻合,能具体、准确地反映论文的基本观点和重要论题。

例1:Acute respiratory distress syndrome in adults: diagnosis, outcomes, long-term sequelae, and management

成人急性呼吸窘迫综合征:诊断、结果、长期后遗症和处理

(2) 简明扼要

用准确、精炼的词汇表达尽可能多的信息,反映研究的性质、内容、对象和方法。

例2:Guidelines for pregnant individuals with monkeypox virus exposure

猴痘病毒暴露的孕妇指南

(3) 便于检索

标题中所用词应尽可能包括论文中的关键词,方便为编制题录索引等二次文献提供检索的特定实用信息。

例3:Early Versus Later Anticoagulation for Stroke with Atrial Fibrillation

房颤卒中早期抗凝与晚期抗凝的比较

1.2 标题的书写

不同学术期刊针对标题的书写格式有着不同的要求和惯例。一般来说,标题的书

写格式有三种：

（1）仅首词的第一个字母和通用的缩略语、人名、地名等专有名词各词的首字母大写，其余均为小写。

例 4：Occupational health hazards among healthcare providers and ancillary staff in Ghana：a scoping review

加纳医护人员及辅助人员的职业健康危害研究：范围综述

（2）每个词的首字母均大写，但一些虚词，如冠词、连词和介词首字母小写。有的期刊要求 4 个字母及以上的虚词首字母也要大写。

例 5：Cardiovascular Safety of Testosterone-Replacement Therapy

睾酮替代疗法的心血管安全性

（3）标题中所有字母均大写。这种格式越来越少，目前只有少部分期刊仍在使用这种所有字母均为大写的标题书写格式，如 *Experimental Oncology* 等。

例 6：ON THE ORIGIN OF LUNG CANCER DEVELOPMENT

肺癌发展的起源

关于标题字数，一般没有具体的限制，需要参考各杂志征稿简则。过长的标题，显得累赘、冗长；过短的标题，所提供的信息量不足。因此，应以是否能够全面反映论文主题为标准。投稿前一定要仔细阅读目标期刊的"作者须知"（Information for Authors 或 Author Center 等），获得更详细的说明。

第二节 标题的语法结构

医学论文的英语标题多由短语构成，包括名词短语、动名词短语和介词短语，少数也采用完整的句子，以陈述句和疑问句居多，陈述句的句尾不用句号，疑问句的句尾保留问号。

2.1 短语型标题

2.1.1 名词短语

这种类型标题最为常见，有名词加介词、名词加分词、名词加同位语、名词加不定式、名词加从句等几种结构。

例 1：Serine and Lipid Metabolism in Macular Disease and Peripheral Neuropathy（名词加介词）

丝氨酸和脂质代谢在黄斑病变和周围神经病变中的作用

例 2：Roxadustat Treatment for Anemia in Patients Undergoing Long-Term Dialysis（名词加分词）

长期透析患者用罗沙司他治疗贫血

例 3：Tumor-associated macrophages: Potential target of natural compounds for management of breast cancer（名词加同位语）

肿瘤相关巨噬细胞：天然化合物治疗乳腺癌的潜在靶点

例 4：C-Reactive Protein Testing to Guide Antibiotic Prescribing for COPD Exacerbations（名词加不定式）

C 反应蛋白检测指导 COPD 加重患者的抗生素处方

例 5：More Evidence That Low-Dose Ionizing Radiation Is Associated with Increased Cancer（名词加从句）

更多证据表明小剂量电离辐射与癌症增加相关

2.1.2　动名词短语

例 6：Saving Thyroids—Overtreatment of Small Papillary Cancers
挽救甲状腺——小乳头状癌的过度治疗
例 7：Using Artificial Intelligence to Predict Atrial Fibrillation
利用人工智能预测心房颤动

2.1.3　介词短语

例 8：After the Storm—A Responsible Path for Genome Editing
风暴过后——探索负责任的基因组编辑之路
例 9：On lymphocyte subpopulation in diabetic mothers at delivery and in their newborn

糖尿病母亲分娩时及其新生儿淋巴细胞亚群研究

2.2　句子型标题

句子型标题以陈述句和疑问句居多，陈述句句尾不用句号，但疑问句句尾仍需保留问号。

2.2.1　陈述句

例 10：Vitamin E Alone Is Ineffective for NASH in Patients with Type 2 Diabetes
维生素 E 单独用药对 2 型糖尿病患者的非酒精性脂肪性肝炎无效
例 11：Leptin attenuates the anti-estrogen effect of tamoxifen in breast cancer
瘦素减弱他莫昔芬在乳腺癌的抗雌激素作用

2.2.2 疑问句

例12：Can Endoscopic Remodeling of the Duodenum Treat Type 2 Diabetes Mellitus?

内镜下十二指肠重塑可否治疗2型糖尿病？

例13：Is High Dietary Calcium Intake Associated with Better Bone Density?

高膳食钙摄入量是否与较好的骨密度相关？

第三节　副标题

副标题是对正标题的补充与说明，以突出论文某方面的内容，如病例数、研究方法等。正副标题之间一般用冒号或破折号分开。常见的副标题主要应用于以下几个方面：

（1）突出病例数或研究时长

例1：Abdominal pain in the emergency room：a study of 176 consecutive cases

腹痛急诊——176例连续病例研究

例2：The FDA Breakthrough-Drug Designation—Four Years of Experience

FDA突破性药物的认定——4年经验

（2）突出研究方法或性质

例3：Leader genes in osteogenesis：a theoretical study

骨形成中的先导基因：一项理论研究

例4：A Fully Magnetically Levitated Left Ventricular Assist Device—Final Report

全磁悬浮左心室辅助装置——最终报告

（3）突出重点内容

例5：Esketamine for Treatment-Resistant Depression—First FDA-Approved Antidepressant in a New Class

艾氯胺酮治疗难治性抑郁症——FDA批准的首款新型抗抑郁药

（4）突出治疗作用，表示同位关系

例6：Prazosin：a new vasodilator used for treatment of hypertension

派唑嗪：一种用于治疗高血压的新型血管扩张剂

（5）提出疑问或选择

例7：Estrogen-Progestin Therapy Elevates Risk for Breast Cancer—Should This

Influence Clinical Practice?

雌激素—孕激素疗法增加乳腺癌风险,这是否会影响临床实践?

（6）表示长篇连载论文各分篇的主题

这种情况一般在副标题前加上罗马数字Ⅰ、Ⅱ、Ⅲ、Ⅳ、Ⅴ等,以示连续性。

例8：Medical treatment of early breast cancer Ⅰ：adjuvant treatment

Medical treatment of early breast cancer Ⅱ：endocrine therapy

Medical treatment of early breast cancer Ⅲ：chemotherapy

Medical treatment of early breast cancer Ⅳ：neoadjuvant treatment

早期乳腺癌的医学治疗（Ⅰ）：辅助治疗

早期乳腺癌的医学治疗（Ⅱ）：内分泌治疗

早期乳腺癌的医学治疗（Ⅲ）：化疗

早期乳腺癌的医学治疗（Ⅳ）：新辅助治疗

第四节　标题常用句式

一个好的标题犹如一篇学术论文的广告,要能起到"画龙点睛"的作用,能够使用最简洁、最恰当的语言表达学术论文的创新点和价值,从而增加读者的好奇心,进一步去阅读和研究论文的具体内容。下面介绍一下标题语言中的省略现象和几种常用的标题句式。

4.1　标题中的省略现象

医学论文英文标题应以简洁为主,重心放在表意的内容词(content words)上,往往省略不表意的功能词(function words)。英文标题中,疾病名称、手术名称或专有名词前一般不用冠词。

例1：Improved Regorafenib Dosing for Refractory Metastatic Colorectal Cancer
改进瑞戈非尼剂量,治疗难治的转移性结直肠癌

例2：Clinical Course and Management of Hypertrophic Cardiomyopathy
肥厚型心肌病的临床病程和治疗

在标题的开头,一些范畴词汇如 Nature of、Studies of、Experience of、Preliminary 等往往可以省略;病例报告和临床科研常用的"心得""体会"在英文标题中往往省略;汉语标题惯用的谦辞,例如"初步"研究、"小"议、"刍"议等对应的英文词汇也往往省略。

例3：

原标题：A preliminary study of anxious and depressive disorders in patients with stroke

修改后：Anxious and depressive disorders in patients with stroke

脑卒中患者焦虑和抑郁性障碍研究

例 4：

原标题：Experience of dendritic cell immunotherapy in ovarian cancer

修改后：Dendritic cell immunotherapy in ovarian cancer

卵巢癌树突状细胞免疫治疗经验

但需注意的是，标题中的"study（研究）"前如带有表明该项研究的特性修饰语时，例如 comparative study（对比性研究）、retrospective study（回顾性研究）、randomized study（随机研究）时，study 不宜省略。

例 5：

Screening for prostate cancer：an updated study

前列腺癌筛查：最新研究

例 6：

Diabetic nephropathy：A retrospective study

糖尿病肾病的回顾性研究

4.2 几种常用的标题句式

4.2.1 药物治疗类常见标题句式

(1) 药物名称＋in / for＋病名

(2) 药物名称＋in the treatment / management of＋病名

(3) 药物名称＋therapy / treatment of＋病名

(4) Treatment of＋病名＋with＋药物名称

(5) Use of ＋药物名称＋in the treatment of＋病名

例 7：HDP-CDV as an alternative for treatment of human herpesvirus-6 infections

治疗人类疱疹病毒-6 感染的替代药物 HDP-CDV

例 8：Telbivudine in the treatment of hepatitis B-associated cryoglobulinemia

替比夫定治疗乙型肝炎相关冷球蛋白血症

例 9：Vancomycin therapy of bacterial meningitis

万古霉素治疗细菌性脑膜炎

例 10：Treatment of carcinoma of uterine cervix with taxol

紫杉醇治疗子宫颈癌

例 11：Use of levodopa in the treatment of Parkinson's disease

左旋多巴在治疗帕金森症中的作用

4.2.2 治疗方法类常见标题句式

（1）治疗方法＋in / for＋病名

（2）治疗方法＋in the treatment / management of＋病名

（3）Treatment of ＋病名＋by / with＋治疗方法

例 12：A neural strategy for directional behaviour

定向行为神经策略

例 13：Pleuropneumonectomy in the management of diffuse malignant mesothelioma of pleura

胸膜肺切除术治疗弥漫性恶性胸膜间皮瘤

例 14：Treatment of intractable ascites in patients with alcoholic cirrhosis by peritoneoveous shunting

腹膜静脉分流术治疗酒精性肝硬化患者顽固性腹水

4.2.3 诊断方法类常见标题句式

（1）诊断方法＋in＋病名

（2）诊断方法＋in the diagnosis of＋病名

（3）Assay / detection of＋某种成分＋in＋病名

（4）Diagnosis of＋病名＋by / with via using＋诊断方法

（5）Application of＋诊断方法＋to the diagnosis of＋病名

例 15：Trypotophan test in stomach cancer

色氨酸试验诊断胃癌

例 16：Enzyme-linked immunosorbent assay（ELLSA） in the diagnosis of amebiasis

酶联免疫吸附法诊断阿米巴病

例 17：Assay of the mineral contents of bone in hepatic cirrhosis patients

肝硬化患者骨矿物质含量检测

例 18：Diagnosis of pulmonary tuberculosis by flexible fiberoptic bronchoscopy

用可曲光学纤维支气管镜检法诊断肺结核

例 19：Application of pulmonary angiography to the diagnosis of acute pneumococcal empyema

肺血管造影图像在诊断急性肺炎双球菌性脓胸中的应用

4.2.4 研究结果类常见标题句式

这种句式经常表现为 Effect / Involvement / Role of A on B

例 20：Effects of nerve growth factor on the neuronal apoptosis after spinal cord injury in rats

神经生长因子对大鼠脊髓损伤后神经元凋亡的影响

例 21：Side effects of phenobarbital and carbamazepine in childhood epilepsy：randomized controlled study

苯巴比妥和卡马西平治疗儿童癫痫的副作用：随机对照研究

第五节 英汉医学论文标题对比

英语和汉语分属不同语系，词法、句式上均有很大区别。英汉语医学论文标题主要在以下几个方面存在着差异。

5.1 范畴词的使用

汉语医学论文标题中的"关于""有关""研究""报告""观察""分析""体会"等无实质性内容的范畴词在英文标题中往往省略，或置于副标题中，以利于编制索引。

例 1：The dynamics of ammonia metabolism in man

人类氨代谢动力学（研究）

例 2：Clinical efficacy of disopyramide in the treatment of cardiac arrhythmias

丙吡胺治疗心律失常的临床疗效（观察）

例 3：Complete Revascularization with Multivessel PCI for Myocardial Infarction

全血运重建与多血管 PCI 心肌梗死（体会）

5.2 as 结构的应用

医学英文论文中，短语型标题使用的比较多，句子型标题也有，但不如短语型标题常见，在需要用谓语或同位语时，常用带 as 的结构表示。

例 4：Tumor angiogenesis as a predictor of recurrence in gastric carcinoma

肿瘤血管生成是胃癌复发的预测因子

例 5：Gastrocolic fistula as a complication of benign gastric ulcer

胃结肠瘘——胃良性溃疡的并发症

例 6：Angiodysplasia as a cause of colonic bleeding in the elderly

血管发育不全是老年人结肠出血的原因之一

例 7：Thyroid cancer as a late consequence of head-neck irradiation

头颈放射的晚期后果：甲状腺癌

5.3 表示关联关系句式的应用

医学英文论文标题中,表达各个概念的词或词组的先后顺序通常借助并列连词 and 来表达,汉语标题中的"关系"一词,也可以直接借助 and、relevance、correlation 等词汇表达,不需专门译出。

例 8:Pesticides and atopic and nonatopic asthma among farm women in the agricultural health study

农业健康研究探讨杀虫剂和农业妇女的过敏性和非过敏性哮喘关系

例 9:Serum uric acid and perioperative and late cardiovascular outcome in patients with suspected or definite Coronary Artery Disease undergoing elective vascular surgery

疑似或确诊的冠状动脉疾病患者选择性血管手术时血清尿酸与围手术期及晚期心血管结局关系研究

例 10:Dihydropiridine calcium-channel blockers and perioperative mortality in aortic aneurysm surgery

二氢吡啶钙通道阻滞剂与主动脉瘤手术围手术期死亡率的关系研究

例 11:Vitamin D and its therapeutic relevance in pulmonary diseases

维生素 D 及其在肺部疾病中的治疗意义

例 12:Clinical Correlation of Intraoperative Neuromonitoring in 319 Individuals Undergoing Posterior Decompression and Fixation of Spine

319 例脊柱后路减压固定术中神经监测的临床相关性

例 13:Clinical relevance of tumour-associated macrophages

肿瘤相关巨噬细胞的临床意义

5.4 病例数的处理

国内外医学期刊对于标题中的病例数采取不同的处理方式。在国外,病例数大多置于副标题中,或在正副标题都不体现,只在摘要或正文中说明。然而,我国医学论文标题,为吸引读者注意,往往将病例数置于正标题中。所以,将汉语标题翻译成英语时最好将病例数置于副标题。

例 14:Fine-needle aspiration cytology of salivary gland:a review of 341 cases

341 例涎腺细针穿刺细胞学检查回顾

例 15:Acute necrotizing enterocolitis in infancy:a review of 64 cases

64 例婴儿急性坏死性小肠结肠炎回顾分析

例 16:Tricuspid valve replacement:clinical analysis of 55 cases

55 例三尖瓣置换术临床分析

第六节 练习巩固

1. 请将下列标题译成汉语。

（1）Therapeutic effect of acupuncture point injection with placental extract in knee osteoarthritis

_____

（2）Diagnostic Use of Base Excess in Acid-Base Disorders

_____

（3）Acupuncture for migraine without aura：a systematic review and meta-analysis

_____

（4）Post-Transplantation Lymphoproliferative Disorders in Adults

_____

（5）Update on Clinical Aspects of Chronic Obstructive Pulmonary Disease

_____

（6）Can menopausal hormone therapy prevent muscle atrophy?

_____

（7）Clinical and Genomic Risk to Guide the Use of Adjuvant Therapy for Breast Cancer

_____

（8）A Randomized Trial of Lymphadenectomy in Patients with Advanced Ovarian Neoplasms

_____

（9）Ambient Particulate Air Pollution and Daily Mortality in 652 Cities

_____

（10）Trial of SAGE-217 in Patients with Major Depressive Disorder

_____

2. 请将下列标题中的介词补充完整。

（1）Catheter Ablation _____ Ventricular Arrhythmias

（2）Are Screen Time and Depression _____ Adolescents Linked?

（3）Effects of exercise training _____ anxiety _____ diabetic rats

（4）Recognition _____ Discoveries _____ DNA Repair

（5）Thrombolysis Guided _____ Perfusion Imaging up _____ 9 Hours _____ Onset _____ Stroke

（6）Comparative effects _____ pharmacological interventions _____ the acute and long-term management _____ insomnia disorder _____ adults

（7）Efficacy and safety _____ abrocitinib _____ dupilumab _____ adults _____ moderate- _____ -severe atopic dermatitis

（8）Complement activation _____ cancer：Effects _____ tumor-associated myeloid cells and immunosuppression

（9）Baseline immunity and impact _____ chemotherapy _____ immune microenvironment _____ cervical cancer

3. 根据下面的信息，编写完整的标题。

（1）incidence，mortality，breast cancer，Asia-Pacific region
亚太地区乳腺癌发病率和死亡率研究

_____

（2）lateral pterygoid muscle，anatomic section，CT
翼外侧肌的解剖切片和 CT 表现研究

_____

（3）progress，intrahepatic，cholangiolithiasis，cholangiocarcinoma
肝内胆管结石合并胆管癌的研究进展

_____

（4）preoperative，intravascular，dezocine，postoperative，pain，laparoscopic cholecystectomy
术前注射内地佐辛可减少腹腔镜胆囊切除术术后疼痛

_____

（5）pathological changes，gastric mucosa，Hpylori eradication，five-year follow up
幽门螺旋杆菌根除后胃黏膜的病理变化：一项为期五年的随访研究

_____

（6）toxicity，concurrent stereotactic chemotherapy，target therapy，immunotherapy，systematic review
同步立体定向化疗和靶向治疗或免疫治疗的毒性研究：系统综述

_____

（7）ultrasonographic value，nodular goiter，thyroid cancer
甲状腺癌结节性甲状腺肿的超声诊断价值

_____

（8）acetylcholine and choline concentration，cerebrospinal fluid，Alzhimer's Disease，vascular dementia

阿尔茨海默病患者和血管性痴呆患者脑脊液中乙酰胆碱和胆碱浓度的差异

（9）diagnostic criteria，viral myocarditis，children

小儿病毒性心肌炎诊断标准

（10）dose-dependent，parathyroid hormone，fracture healing，bone formation，mice

甲状旁腺激素对小鼠骨折愈合和骨形成的剂量依赖效应

4. 请将下列标题译成英语。

（1）老年男性睾酮替代疗法的安全性

（2）妊娠早期诊断的妊娠期糖尿病治疗

（3）补充微量营养素以降低心血管风险

（4）长期全身性皮质类固醇暴露：系统性文献综述

（5）肿瘤微环境的临床相关性：免疫细胞、血管和小鼠模型

第三章　摘　要

摘要犹如学术论文的一扇窗口，通过阅读摘要，读者可获得相关论文的主要观点和结论，明白论文的主要创新点，从而决定是否需要继续阅读全文。因此，论文的摘要必需清楚、简明、要点齐全而不能笼统、含糊，一篇好的摘要甚至可以弥补正文概述中的不足。总体而言，医学学术论文的摘要应具有简明性、完整性、科学性和准确性几大特征。

第一节　摘要的分类

按摘要性质，医学论文摘要大致可以分为以下四类：报道性摘要（informative abstract）、指示性摘要（indicative abstract）、报道—指示性摘要（informative-indicative abstract）和结构式摘要（structured abstract）。结构式摘要已成为国际期刊普遍采用的摘要模式。

1.1　报道性摘要

报道性摘要（informative abstract）也称资料性摘要，属于传统型摘要的一种。这类摘要往往是一篇完整的短文，内容包括研究目的、研究材料和方法、研究结果、研究结论等，层层展开，能较完整地概括正文的主要内容。

例 1：The exposure of cells, tissues and extracellular matrix to harmful reactive species causes a cascade of reactions and induces activation of multiple internal defence mechanisms (enzymatic or non-enzymatic) that provide removal of reactive species and their derivatives. The non-enzymatic antioxidants are represented by molecules characterized by the ability to rapidly inactivate radicals and oxidants. This paper focuses on the major intrinsic non-enzymatic antioxidants，including metal binding proteins(MBPs), glutathione (GSH)，uric acid (UA)，melatonin (MEL)，bilirubin (BIL) and polyamines (PAs).

[Excerpted from Endogenous non-enzymatic antioxidants in the human body. *Advances in Medical Sciences*，2018，63(1)：68 - 78.]

这一段报道性摘要一共只有 3 句话，但逻辑清晰，句子前后照应，层层展开，一步步引导读者关注研究的重点内容。第一句首先介绍研究背景,指出两种防御机制——酶或非酶抗氧化剂的激活条件。第二句将范围缩小,只讨论非酶抗氧化剂的表达方式。第三句指出本文的研究内容和范围,即对一些非酶抗氧化剂的重点研究。

1.2 指示性摘要

指示性摘要(indicative abstract)也称说明性摘要、描述性摘要,它的特点是一般不涉及实质性材料,只做原则性介绍,内容和结构一般比较简单,只说明论文的研究主题而不具体介绍研究方法和结果。指示性摘要往往语句不长,多用于病例报告、综述、会议报告等。

例 2:An 81-year-old man presents to the ER with an acute ischemic stroke; IV thrombolytic therapy is recommended. Administered as a therapeutic agent within 4. 5 hours after stroke, tissue plasminogen activator has been shown to improve neurologic outcomes.

这是一段典型的指示性摘要,只有 2 句话,内容和结构均较简单。通过第一句对病例的简单介绍,直接过渡到第二句,点明了研究的价值所在,即组织纤溶酶原激活剂(tissue plasminogen activator)能够改善神经功能结局。这篇摘要没有涉及具体的研究方法和研究过程等内容。

1.3 报道—指示性摘要

报道—指示性摘要(informative-indicative abstract)是一种报道与指示性相结合的综合性摘要。它的特点是对文献中信息价值较高、重要的部分以报道性形式表达,而对其余次要部分以指示性表述。

例 3:Thyroid disorders are the most common endocrine diseases and affect a large segment of the population. Most of the thyroid diseases are autoimmune in nature and can be broadly grouped into two categories:one mediated by autoimmune responses to the thyroglobulin (i. e. Hashimoto's thyroiditis), and the other mediated by autoimmunity to the thyrotropin receptor (primarily Graves' disease). Although patients with autoimmune thyroid diseases exhibit immune responses against a number of thyroid antigens, such as thyroglobulin, thyrotropin receptor and thyroid peroxidase, responses directed against a specific antigen appear to play an important role in the disease pathogenesis. For example, Hashimoto's thyroiditis is primarily mediated by T cell responses directed toward the thyroglobulin receptor, whereas Graves' disease is mediated by antibodies directed against the thyrotropin receptor. In this review we will focus on thyroid diseases mediated by autoimmune responses to the thyrotropin receptor.

〔Excerpted from Autoimmunity to the thyroid stimulating hormone receptor. *Advances in Neuroimmunology*，1996，6(4)：347－357.〕

这一段报道—指示性摘要对研究背景描述得较为详细，首先介绍了甲状腺疾病的本质及两种分类，随后分别介绍两种甲状腺疾病的发病机制，强调特异性抗原引起的免疫反应在发病机制中的重要性。最后一句过渡到本文研究的主要内容，即关注由促甲状腺激素受体的自身免疫反应介导的甲状腺疾病。

1.4 结构式摘要

结构式摘要（structured abstract）是目前国际学术期刊普遍采用的摘要模式，即摘要的撰写要遵循一定的格式要求，并由明确的提示词表明各部分的内容，作者需要按照各部分的内容提示词将摘要呈现出来，便于读者阅读。一般来说，结构式摘要主要包含以下几个方面的内容：

背景（Background）

目的（Objective/Purpose/Aim/Introduction）

方法（Methods）

结果（Results/Findings）

结论（Conclusions）

有的杂志要求摘要只需包括后面四个部分，即目的、方法、结果和讨论，有的杂志只要求对背景、结果和结论三个部分进行介绍，还有的杂志不限于以上这些部分，要求更多、更详细的摘要内容。具体要求需仔细阅读各种期刊的作者须知。下面举例说明结构式摘要的格式要求和基本特征。

例 4：

BACKGROUND

The hemoglobin threshold for transfusion of red cells in patients with acute gastrointestinal bleeding is controversial. We compared the efficacy and safety of a restrictive transfusion strategy with those of a liberal transfusion strategy.

METHODS

We enrolled 921 patients with severe acute upper gastrointestinal bleeding and randomly assigned 461 of them to a restrictive strategy (transfusion when the hemoglobin level fell below 7 g per deciliter) and 460 to a liberal strategy (transfusion when the hemoglobin fell below 9 g per deciliter). Randomization was stratified according to the presence or absence of liver cirrhosis.

RESULTS

A total of 225 patients assigned to the restrictive strategy (51%), as compared with 61 assigned to the liberal strategy (14%), did not receive transfusions (P< 0.001). The probability of survival at 6 weeks was higher in the restrictive-strategy group than in the liberal-strategy group (95% vs. 91%; hazard ratio for death with restrictive strategy, 0. 55; 95% confidence interval [CI], 0. 33 to 0. 92; P=0. 02). Further bleeding occurred in 10% of the patients in the restrictive-strategy group as compared with 16% of the patients in the liberal-strategy group (P=0. 01), and adverse events occurred in 40% as compared with 48% (P=0. 02). The probability of survival was slightly higher with the restrictive strategy than with the liberal strategy in the subgroup of patients who had bleeding associated with a peptic ulcer (hazard ratio, 0. 70; 95% CI, 0. 26 to 1. 25) and was significantly higher in the subgroup of patients with cirrhosis and Child-Pugh class A or B disease (hazard ratio, 0. 30; 95% CI, 0. 11 to 0. 85), but not in those with cirrhosis and Child-Pugh class C disease (hazard ratio, 1. 04; 95% CI, 0. 45 to 2. 37). Within the first 5 days, the portal-pressure gradient increased significantly in patients assigned to the liberal strategy (P=0. 03) but not in those assigned to the restrictive strategy.

CONCLUSIONS

As compared with a liberal transfusion strategy, a restrictive strategy significantly improved outcomes in patients with acute upper gastrointestinal bleeding.

[Excerpted from Transfusion Strategies for Acute Upper Gastrointestinal Bleeding. *N Engl J Med*, 2013, 368: 11 - 21.]

这篇结构式摘要选自《新英格兰医学杂志》(*New England Journal of Medicine*)。在该杂志的"preparation instructions"中,对"abstract"的要求是这样的:"Provide an abstract of no more than 250 words with four labeled paragraphs containing the following: 1. Background: Problem being addressed in the study; 2. Methods: How the study was performed; 3. Results: Salient results; 4. Conclusions: What the authors conclude from study results."从这里可以清楚地看出摘要的各组成部分,即背景、方法、结果和结论的具体写作内容。

这篇摘要的"背景"部分,作者首先说明现在存在争议的问题,然后交代本文针对这个争议所做的研究。在"方法"部分,作者使用两个句子介绍了研究对象、数量和分组标准。接下来,作者重点描述了"结果"部分,就生存率、再出血率、不良事件发生率等指标进行了对比,共使用五个句子,以此突出研究的新发现。"结论"部分只用了一句话概述该研究所得到的最终结论。

1.5 其他结构式摘要

还有一种结构式摘要包含的内容更多,一些国际知名杂志如《英国医学杂志》(*British Medical Journal*, BMJ)和《美国医学学会杂志》(*The Journal of the American Medical Association*, JAMA)刊登的论文摘要主要包括以下几个要素:

目的（Objective/Purpose）

设计（Design）

背景 （Setting）

对象 （Patients，Participants or Subjects）

处置方法 （Interventions）

主要测定项目 （Main Outcome Measures）

结果 （Results）

结论 （Conclusion）

有时候以上小标题名称会有所更改，但基本内容不变。

例 5：

Objective

Low neighbourhood socioeconomic status （NSES） has been linked to a higher risk of overweight/obesity，irrespective of the individual's own socioeconomic status. No meta-analysis study has been done on the association. Thus，this study was done to synthesize the existing evidence on the association of NSES with overweight，obesity and body mass index （BMI）.

Design

Systematic review and meta-analysis.

Data sources

PubMed，Embase，Scopus，Cochrane Library，Web of Sciences and Google Scholar databases were searched for articles published until 25 September 2019.

Eligibility criteria

Epidemiological studies，both longitudinal and cross-sectional ones，which examined the link of NSES to overweight，obesity or BMI，were included.

Data extraction and synthesis

Data extraction was done by two reviewers，working independently. The methodological quality of included studies was assessed using the Newcastle-Ottawa Scale for the observational studies. The summary estimates of the relationships of NSES with overweight，obesity and BMI statuses were calculated with random-effects meta-analysis models. Heterogeneity was assessed by Cochran's Q and I2 statistics. Subgroup analyses were done by age categories，continents，study designs and NSES measures. Publication bias was assessed by visual inspection of funnel plots and Egger's regression test.

Result

A total of 21 observational studies，covering 1 244 438 individuals，were included in this meta-analysis. Low NSES，compared with high NSES，was found to be associated with a 31% higher odds of overweight （pooled OR 1. 31，95% CI 1. 16 to

1.47，p<0.001），a 45％ higher odds of obesity（pooled OR 1.45，95％ CI 1.21 to 1.74，p<0.001）and a 1.09 kg/m^2 increase in mean BMI（pooled beta＝1.09，95％ CI 0.67 to 1.50，p<0.001）.

Conclusion

NSES disparity might be contributing to the burden of overweight/obesity. Further studies are warranted，including whether addressing NSES disparity could reduce the risk of overweight/obesity.

〔Excerpted from Neighbourhood socioeconomic status and overweight/obesity: a systematic review and meta-analysis of epidemiological studies. *BMJ* Open，2019，9(11):e028238.〕

这篇摘要选自《英国医学杂志》(*British Medical Journal*，*BMJ*)，在该杂志的"Submission Guidelines"中明确指出摘要应该是"a structured abstract"，最多 300 个词，包含以下几个部分：Objectives、Design、Setting、Participants、Interventions、Primary and Secondary Outcome Measures、Results and Conclusions。由于这篇论文是系统性综述和荟萃分析类文章，摘要的具体小标题略有变动。在"目的"部分，作者共使用三句话，前两句交代了研究背景，使用了现在完成时，最后一句交代了本文的研究目的，使用了过去时；在"设计"部分，点明了本研究属于系统综述和荟萃分析；紧接着在"数据来源"部分，作者说明研究数据从哪些方面获取；在"资格标准"中，说明研究数据入选的标准；在"数据提取和合成"中，作者详细交代了研究方法；在"结果"部分，作者使用过去时交代了本次研究所得的结果；最终在"结论"的两句话中，作者首先使用了模糊限制词"might"，表明作者对本次研究结论的谨慎态度，然后在第二句中借助"further studies are warranted"表达作者对未来相关研究的期望。

第二节　摘要的语言特征与时态运用

2.1　摘要中第一人称的表达

摘要中经常会出现"我"或"我们"这一概念，以描述研究目的或研究方法，例如"我们的目的是……""我们收集了……"等句型。在用英文表达时，就有主动语态或被动语态的选用问题。与其他类型的科技论文相似，英语医学学术论文中使用被动语态的句子占大多数，这种表达方式一方面避免单一使用主动语态的沉闷、乏味，一方面突出了动作对象的主体地位，从而体现了科技论文客观、公正的科学原则。然而，也有一种观点认为科技论文中主动语态的使用会拉近作者与读者的距离，显得语气自然、亲切。因此，主动语态或被动语态的使用并无统一标准，应视语言表达的上下文和具体情况而定。下面具体分析医学学术论文摘要中需要表述第一人称"我"或"我们"这一概念时的几种处理方法。

2.1.1　使用主动语态和复数第一人称代词"we"表达

在报道性摘要中,当描述"编者、研究者"等概念时,常用第一人称代词复数形式,即"we"表达。

例1:Here we report the first case of two siblings with neurofibromatosis type 1 (NF1),who suffered an acute ischemic stroke.

我们报道了兄妹两位中第一位患1型神经纤维瘤病(NF1)的患者,其患急性缺血性中风。

例2:We aimed to systematically review the present literature to determine the follow-up rates of large cohorts/registries of total joint arthroplasty patients and to identify factors associated with successful collection of PROMs.

我们旨在系统回顾现有文献,以确定全关节置换术患者的随访率,并确定与成功收集 PROMs 相关的因素。

2.1.2　用被动语态表达

被动语态表达方式虽然没有明显指出动作的执行者,但读者可从上下文推断出动作的执行者。目前简便而又不至于引起歧义的被动语态表达方式在英语医学论文中还是非常普遍的。

例3:Complete blood count blood tests were conducted on nineteen Ironman triathletes before and after an Ironman triathlon to characterize changes in hematological parameters and the effect on Athlete Biological Passport (ABP) interpretation, as it was hypothesized that plasma volume (PV) changes may result in the presentation of atypical ABP profiles.

因为有假设认为血浆容量(PV)的变化可能导致非典型运动员生物护照(ABP)特征的出现,我们在铁人三项比赛前后对 19 名铁人三项运动员进行了全血细胞计数血液测试,以证实血液参数的变化和对 ABP 解释的影响。

例4:Daily data on mortality and air pollution were collected from 652 cities in 24 countries or regions.

我们每天从 24 个国家和地区的 652 个城市收集死亡率和空气污染数据。

2.1.3　以 results、report、study 等作主语

在英语医学论文中,作者的研究结果、研究论文(this study、this report、the results)等也可以替代人称第一代词 I 或 we,其中以 the results 最为常见。

例5:Therefore, the current study focused on the investigation of in vitro and in vivo metabolic fate of abemaciclib using high resolution mass spectrometry.

因此,我们目前的研究集中在使用高分辨率质谱技术研究阿贝西利(abemaciclib,一种用于治疗乳腺癌的药物)的体外和体内代谢过程。

例6:These results offer a characterized timeline of hematological changes and expected plasma volume(PV) shifting following an Ironman triathlon providing important data for the reliable interpretation of Athlete Biological Passport(ABP) profiles in this field.

这些结果提供了铁人三项赛后血液学变化和预期血浆容量变化的特征性时间表,为该领域运动员生物护照资料的可靠解释提供了重要数据。

2.2 摘要中的时态运用

英语医学论文的特定题材和文体特征约束了摘要中各部分的时态运用。作者通过运用不同的动词时态,向读者表明哪些是研究前已做的工作,哪些是研究过程中所做的工作,哪些是研究结束后得到的暂时性结果,以及哪些是研究结束后得到的较为客观真实、可被普遍推广的结果。这些内容都与特定时态的运用紧密相关。下面逐一分析英语医学论文摘要中的常用时态。

(1)介绍背景通常采用一般现在时和现在完成时,表明在论文写作时的当时情况或强调过去的行为对现在的影响。

例7:Acute coronary syndrome(ACS) is the leading cause of death in developing and developed countries, yet assessing the risk of its development remains challenging. Several lines of evidence indicate that small, dense low-density lipoproteins(sd-LDL) are associated with increased cardiovascular disease risk.

急性冠状动脉综合征是发展中国家和发达国家的主要致死因素,然而评估其发展风险仍然具有挑战性。一些证据表明,小而致密的低密度脂蛋白与心血管疾病风险增加有关。

例8:Abemaciclib is approved by US Food and Drug Administration in 2015 to have an advanced treatment for metastatic breast cancer. Identification and characterization of limited numbers of abemaciclib metabolites have been reported in the literature.

2015年,美国食品药品监督管理局批准使用药物阿贝西利对转移性乳腺癌症进行晚期治疗。文献中已经报道了阿贝西利代谢物的鉴定和表征,但数量有限。

(2)介绍研究目的或意图时,使用一般过去时,以表明研究前所确定的目标,而介绍本文目的时,谓语动词通常采用一般现在时或 be to do 结构。

例9:This study was performed to evaluate whether pretreatment Hgb less than 13 g/dL was correlated with treatment outcome in patients with advanced HNC treated with a uniform regimen of RT/CCT.

本研究旨在评估在接受统一 RT/CCT 方案治疗的晚期 HNC 患者中，治疗前血红蛋白低于 13g/dl 是否与治疗结果相关。

例 10：Here, in this review, we emphasize the effect of physicochemical properties of nanocarriers on their interactions with the biological milieu. The review will discuss in depth, how modulating the physicochemical properties would influence a drug nanocarrier's behavior in vivo and the mechanisms underlying these effects. The goal of this review is to summarize the design considerations based on these properties and to provide a conceptual template for achieving improved therapeutic efficacy with enhanced patient compliance.

在本综述中，我们强调纳米载体的物理化学性质对其与生物环境相互作用的影响。该综述将深入讨论物理化学性质的调节如何影响药物纳米载体在体内的行为以及这些影响背后的机制。本综述的目的是总结基于这些特性的设计考虑因素，并提供一个概念模板，在患者较高依从性的情况下提高治疗效果。

（3）介绍研究方法、过程时，通常只用一般过去时。

例 11：Initially, vulnerable sites of metabolism were predicted by Xenosite web predictor tool. Later, in vitro metabolites were identified from pooled rat liver microsomes, rat S9 fractions and human liver microsomes. Finally, in vivo metabolites have been detected in plasma, urine and feces matrix of male Sprague-Dawley rats.

最初，我们用 Xenosite 网络预测工具预测代谢的易受攻击部位。随后，从汇集的大鼠肝微粒体、大鼠 S9 级部分和人肝微粒体中鉴定出体外代谢物。最后，我们在雄性 Sprague-Dawley 大鼠的血浆、尿液和粪便基质中检测到体内代谢物。

例 12：Baseline characteristics of 121 patients with acute coronary syndrome (ACS) and 172 healthy controls were obtained. Plasma sd-LDL-C (small, dense low-density lipoproteins concentration) was measured using homogeneous assay, and the proportion of sd-LDL-C in LDL-C was detected.

实验中，我们获得了 121 例急性冠状动脉综合征患者和 172 例健康对照者的基线特征，并用均相分析法测量血浆中的 sd-LDL-C 及其在 LDL-C 中的比例。

（4）描述论文中的主要观察结果、陈述某一特定结果时，使用一般过去时。

例 13：There was gender and age effect on the sd-LDL-C concentration and sd-LDL-C/LDL-C ratio among healthy subjects. Elevated sd-LDL-C concentrations and sd-LDL-C/LDL-C ratio were observed in ACS patients with unstable angina pectoris (UAP), non-ST-segment elevation myocardial infarction (NSTEMI), and ST-segment elevation myocardial infarction (STEMI) compared with healthy controls $(P<.05)$.

健康受试者的性别和年龄对 sd-LDL-C 浓度和 sd-LDL-C/LDL-C 比率有影响。与健康对照组相比,患有不稳定型心绞痛、非 ST 段抬高型心肌梗死和 ST 段抬高型心肌梗死的急性冠脉综合征患者的 sd-LDL-C 浓度和 sd-LDL-C/LDL-C 比值升高(P<0.05)。

例 14:Abemaciclib was metabolized via hydroxylation, N-oxidation, N-dealkylation, oxidative deamination followed by reduction and sulfate conjugation. In the human liver microsomes, maximum numbers of metabolites (11 metabolites) were observed and from which M7, M8, M9 and M11 were human specific.

阿贝西利通过羟基化、氮氧化、氮脱烷基、氧化脱氨,然后还原和硫酸盐结合进行代谢。在人肝微粒体中,我们观察到最大数量的代谢物(11 种代谢物),其中 M7、M8、M9 和 M11 是人类特异性的。

(5)摘要中结论部分的时态应用。结论部分是作者对所得结果的评语,乃写作时作者所持观点,无论结论是肯定的还是否定的,谓语动词都用一般现在时。但也有用过去时表述结论的。从英语修辞学上说,过去时和现在时表述不同的时间及影响等概念,前者表示作者认为该结论不具普遍性,后者表示作者认为该结论具有普遍性。

例 15:Two automated alerts directing clinic personnel and families to have adolescents self-report significantly and sustainably improved younger adolescent self-reporting on electronic patient-generated health data instruments.

指导诊所人员和家庭成员让青少年在电子健康数据仪器上进行自我报告的两台自动警报设备,可显著且持续提高青少年的自我报告能力。

例 16:Readily available clinical variables do not meaningfully improve the prediction of pediatric readmissions and would be unlikely to enhance case-mix adjustment unless their distributions varied widely across hospitals.

现成的临床变量并不能有效地改善儿科再入院的预测,也不太可能加强病例组合调整,除非它们在医院之间的分布差异很大。

此外,结论部分作者会经常使用一些情态动词等模糊限制语表达对结论的委婉看法和不确定态度,让读者感觉易于接受。

例 17:The sd-LDL-C/LDL-C ratio may be associated with an increased risk of developing ACS in Chinese population.

Sd-LDL-C/LDL-C 比率可能与中国人群患急性冠脉综合征的风险增加有关。

例 18:The e-SBI seems to have better potential than ordinary alcohol screening and intervention for implementation into routine emergency departments due to its simplicity and low time consumption.

由于其简便性和低耗时性,电子 SBI 似乎比普通酒精筛查和干预更有潜力,可用于常规应急部门。

第三节 摘要各部分常用句型

英语医学论文的摘要往往只包含几个句子,但这些句子都有明确的含义和作用,使得整个摘要内容连贯、意思完整。下面分析一下结构式摘要中各部分常用句型。

3.1 "目的"部分常用句型

研究论文的目的可以直接借用动词不定式短语来引导,这种句式简单明了,十分常见。

例 1:<u>To review</u> the current knowledge of persistent visual loss after nonocular surgeries under general anesthesia.

以回顾全身麻醉下非眼科手术后持续性视力丧失的现有知识。

例 2:<u>To evaluate</u> the most appropriate surgical method of hysterectomy (abdominal, vaginal, or laparoscopic) for women with benign disease.

本文评估对妇女良性疾病行子宫切除术(腹式、阴道式或腹腔镜式)的最佳手术方案。

也有的研究论文的目的采用非不定式引导,通常借助下列常用词和句型:

- the purpose/aim/of this study/investigation was to ...
- the present study was undertaken to ...
- attempts were made to ...

例 3:<u>This study was designed to</u> evaluate the long-term cardiovascular benefit of bezafibrate therapy in coronary heart disease patients enrolled in the BIP (Bezafibrate Infarction Prevention) trial.

本研究旨在评估苯扎贝特治疗对参与 BIP(苯扎贝特梗死预防)试验的冠心病患者带来的长期心血管益处。

例 4:<u>The goal of this study was intended to</u> know the process of tissue response and regeneration in the palato-maxillary suture under tensile forces.

本研究的目的是了解张力作用下腭—上颌缝合的组织反应和再生过程。

3.2 "方法"部分常用句型

英语医学论文摘要中的方法(Methods)包括两部分内容:研究对象和研究方法。研究对象的一般情况,如性别、年龄、诊断、是否为特殊群体等需要先交代清楚,研究方法的具体内容,如随机分组、对照、双盲、采用的干预方法或技术名称、给药途径和剂量等需要明确表达。

3.2.1 研究对象的描述

医学研究中涉及的受试者、参与者、健康对照组等多是群体,且分组进行,表达分组的常用句型有:

- be randomly divided/categorized/separated/allocated/stratified into ... groups
- be assigned to ...

例5:A total of 198 patients underwent randomization, and 194 were included in the analysis. After adjudication, 60 cases of ventilator-associated pneumonia were confirmed, including 51 of early ventilator-associated pneumonia. The incidence of early ventilator-associated pneumonia was lower with antibiotic prophylaxis than with placebo (19 patients [19%] vs. 32 [34%]; hazard ratio, 0.53; 95% confidence interval, 0.31 to 0.92; P=0.03). No significant differences between the antibiotic group and the control group were observed with respect to the incidence of late ventilator-associated pneumonia (4% and 5%, respectively), the number of ventilator-free days (21 days and 19 days), ICU length of stay (5 days and 8 days if patients were discharged and 7 days and 7 days if patients had died), and mortality at day 28 (41% and 37%). At day 7, no increase in resistant bacteria was identified. Serious adverse events did not differ significantly between the two groups.

共有198名患者接受了随机分组,其中194名纳入分析。经裁定,确诊60例呼吸机相关性肺炎,包括51例早期呼吸机相关性肺炎。抗生素预防组的早期呼吸机相关性肺炎的发生率低于安慰剂组[19名(19%):32名(34%);风险比0.53;95%置信区间,0.31-0.92;P=0.03]。抗生素组和对照组在晚期呼吸机相关性肺炎的发生率(分别为4%和5%)、无呼吸机天数(21天和19天)、重症监护病房的住院时间(出院时为5天和8天,死亡时为7天和7天)以及第28天的死亡率(41%和37%)方面没有观察到显著差异。在第7天,没有发现耐药细菌增加。两组之间的严重不良反应没有显著差异。

这篇摘要中的研究方法部分详细描述了研究对象分组的情况,使用了过去时态。其中涉及很多常用的短语:

- undergo randomization 接受随机分组
- significant differences 显著差异
- serious adverse events 严重不良反应

例6:In the Diabetes Control and Complications Trial (DCCT), 1441 persons with type 1 diabetes were randomly assigned to 6.5 years of intensive diabetes therapy aimed at achieving near-normal glucose concentrations or to conventional diabetes therapy aimed at preventing hyperglycemic symptoms.

在糖尿病控制和并发症试验(DCCT)中,1 441 名 1 型糖尿病患者被随机分配到 6.5 年强化糖尿病治疗组(旨在达到接近正常的葡萄糖浓度)或常规糖尿病治疗组(旨在预防高血糖症状)。

也有的句子并没有出现明显"分组"的提示语,以间接的方式表达分组情况。

例 7:Either intravenous amoxicillin-clavulanate (at doses of 1 g and 200 mg, respectively) or placebo was administered three times a day for 2 days, starting less than 6 hours after the cardiac arrest.

从心脏骤停后不到 6 小时开始,每天三次静脉注射阿莫西林-克拉维酸盐(剂量分别为 1 g 和 200 mg)或安慰剂,持续 2 天。

3.2.2 研究方法的描述

不同医学研究课题采用的研究方法不同,相应的英语表述方式也有差异。常用英文表达"方法"的主要句式有:

- with/by/by means of/using/employing+研究方法

例 8:Serum creatinine levels were measured annually throughout the course of the two studies. The glomerular filtration rate(GFR)was estimated with the use of the Chronic Kidney Disease Epidemiology Collaboration formula.

两项研究的整个过程中,每年测定一次血清肌酐水平。应用慢性肾病流行病学合作公式估算肾小球滤过率(GFR)。

3.3 "结果"部分常用句型

英语医学论文摘要中的结果部分是对研究目的及其所提出的问题的直接回答,是作者得到的第一手资料,描述必须完整、清晰、客观、准确,不能带有任何主观色彩,也不要掺杂前人或他人的研究成果。"结果"部分常用句式中有的直接以"the result of"或"results"做主语引导。

例 9:As a result of Fast Track, the Emergency Department waiting area is less congested and staff moral has increased. A further consequence of Fast Track is that nurses are providing more advanced clinical services to patients.

由于有了快速通道,急诊科的候诊区不再拥挤,工作人员的道德水平得到了提高。快速通道的另一个结果是护士为病人提供更先进的临床服务。

例 10:Among 4392 participants, baseline metabolic disorders (fasting glucose, systolic and diastolic blood pressures) were significantly associated with poorer Cognitive Abilities Screening Instrument (CASI), Digit Symbol Coding(DSC), and Digit Span(DS) scores measured 10 years later. Increases in blood pressure were associated with lower cognitive performance. <u>Results did not differ by</u> race/ethnicity and were stronger among those without the APOE ε4 allele.

在 4 392 名参与者中,基线代谢紊乱(空腹血糖、收缩压和舒张压)与 10 年后测量的认知能力筛查工具、数字符号编码和数字跨度评分较低显著相关。血压升高与认知能力下降有关。结果没有显示种族/民族差异,在没有 APOE ε4 等位基因的人群中更明显。

也有的以"case""specimen""sample""findings"等引导。

例 11:<u>Findings suggest that</u> provider attire is a potential source of pathogenic bacterial transmission in health care settings. However, data confirming a direct link between provider attire and health care-associated infections remain limited. Suggestions outlined in this article may serve as a guideline to reduce the spread of bacterial pathogens, including MDROs, that have the potential to precipitate hospital-acquired infections.

研究结果表明,医护人员的着装是卫生保健机构中致病菌传播的一个潜在来源。然而,证实医疗服务人员着装与医疗相关感染之间存在直接联系的数据仍然有限。本文提出的建议可作为指导方针,以减少包括多药耐药菌(Multiple Drug Resistant Organism,MDRO)在内的细菌病原体传播,其有可能造成医院获得性感染。

例 12:<u>No significant between-group differences were observed</u> for other key clinical variables, such as ventilator-free days and mortality at day 28.

其他关键临床变量,如无呼吸机天数和第 28 天死亡率,未观察到组间显著差异。

例 13:<u>An inverse relationship was noted</u> between efflux capacity and carotid intima-media thickness both before and after adjustment for the HDL cholesterol level.

在调整 HDL 胆固醇水平前后,胆固醇流出量与颈动脉内膜中层厚度之间均呈反比关系。

3.4 "结论"部分常用句型

"结论"部分(Conclusion)是对整个研究及其结果做出的概况、分析、比较和评价,在整篇摘要中起着画龙点睛的作用,应该进行逻辑清晰、精炼完整的描述。"结论"部分常用句型形式多种多样,常见的主要有:

• Our results/findings/data/observation/analysis/experiment(s)/investigation showed/confirmed/indicated/demonstrated/suggested/illustrated/revealed/pointed out that ...

例 14:<u>These results show that</u> marijuana use motives are an important part of understanding the frequency of marijuana use and the development of marijuana use problems. <u>These results may have implications for</u> intervention development and public policy.

这些结果表明,大麻使用动机是了解大麻使用频率和大麻使用问题发展的重要部分。这些结果可能会对干预发展和公共政策产生影响。

例 15：<u>We have discovered and validated</u> a new single saliva biomarker, lactoferrin, which in our cross-sectional investigation perfectly discriminates clinically diagnosed amnestic mild cognitive impairment（aMCI）and Alzheimer's disease（AD）patients from a cognitively healthy control group.

我们发现并验证了一种新的单一唾液生物标记物——乳铁蛋白,在我们的横断面调查中,它将临床诊断为遗忘型轻度认知障碍患者、阿尔茨海默病患者与认知健康的对照组完全区分开来。

需要注意的是,"结论"部分中运用的动词时态反映出作者对其结论的态度和观点。如果作者认为其结论具有普遍性,常用一般现在时表示。

例 16：Despite the characteristic striatum-first pattern，the global rate of amyloid accumulation <u>differs by</u> pre-existing amyloid burden and <u>precedes</u> atrophy or dementia in the DS population，similar to general AD progression.

尽管具有典型的纹状体优先模式,但淀粉样蛋白总体累积率因先前存在的淀粉样蛋白负荷而异,并且在退行性痴呆人群中先于萎缩或痴呆,类似于一般阿尔茨海默病的进展。

例 17：The Amsterdam IADL Questionnaire（A-IADL-Q）short version（A-IADL-Q-SV）<u>consists of</u> 30 items and <u>has maintained</u> the psychometric quality of the original A-IADL-Q. As such, the A-IADL-Q-SV <u>is a concise measure of</u> functional decline.

阿姆斯特丹 IADL 问卷（A-IADL-Q）简写版（A-IADL-Q-SV）由 30 个项目组成,并保持了原始 A-IADL-Q 的心理测量质量。因此,A-IADL-Q-SV 是功能衰退的简明衡量标准。

如果作者认为该结论只为研究结束时得出的结论,并不具备普遍性和推广性,常用一般过去时表示。

此外,前文也有所提及,即如果作者想表达对本研究的预期效果或展望,或是委婉的看法或建议时,可以借助情态动词或 be＋to do 形式。

例 18：Although further studies are needed，the results indicate that lavender extract improves memory and learning，and <u>might be</u> beneficial in patients with these disorders，particularly the patients suffering pain.

尽管还需要进一步的研究,但结果表明,薰衣草提取物能改善记忆和学习,对患这些疾病的患者,尤其是遭受疼痛折磨的患者来说可能是有益的。

第四节　练习巩固

1. 阅读下面论文摘要,分析其结构特征。

BACKGROUND

E-cigarettes are commonly used in attempts to stop smoking, but evidence is limited regarding their effectiveness as compared with that of nicotine products approved as smoking-cessation treatments.

METHODS

We randomly assigned adults attending U. K. National Health Service stop-smoking services to either nicotine-replacement products of their choice, including product combinations, provided for up to 3 months, or an e-cigarette starter pack (a second-generation refillable e-cigarette with one bottle of nicotine e-liquid [18 mg per milli-liter]), with a recommendation to purchase further e-liquids of the flavor and strength of their choice. Treatment included weekly behavioral support for at least 4 weeks. The primary outcome was sustained abstinence for 1 year, which was validated biochemically at the final visit. Participants who were lost to follow-up or did not provide biochemical validation were considered to not be abstinent. Secondary outcomes included participant-reported treatment usage and respiratory symptoms.

RESULTS

A total of 886 participants underwent randomization. The 1-year abstinence rate was 18. 0% in the e-cigarette group, as compared with 9. 9% in the nicotine-replacement group (relative risk, 1. 83; 95% confidence interval [CI], 1. 30 to 2. 58; $P<0.001$). Among participants with 1-year abstinence, those in the e-cigarette group were more likely than those in the nicotine-replacement group to use their assigned product at 52 weeks (80% [63 of 79 participants] vs. 9% [4 of 44 participants]). Overall, throat or mouth irritation was reported more frequently in the e-cigarette group (65. 3%, vs. 51. 2% in the nicotine-replacement group) and nausea more frequently in the nicotine-replacement group (37. 9%, vs. 31. 3% in the e-cigarette group). The e-cigarette group reported greater declines in the incidence of cough and phlegm production from baseline to 52 weeks than did the nicotine-replacement group (relative risk for cough, 0. 8; 95% CI, 0. 6 to 0. 9; relative risk for phlegm, 0. 7; 95% CI, 0. 6 to 0. 9). There were no significant between-group differences in the incidence of wheezing or shortness of breath.

CONCLUSIONS

E-cigarettes were more effective for smoking cessation than nicotine-replacement therapy, when both products were accompanied by behavioral support.

2. 分析下列摘要的结构,并用括号里词汇的适当形式填空。

Background

Apixaban, an oral, direct factor Xa inhibitor, may reduce the risk of 1._____ (recur) ischemic events when 2._____ (add) to antiplatelet therapy after an acute coronary syndrome.

Methods

We 3._____ (conduct) a 4._____ (random), double-blind, placebo- 5._____ (control) clinical trial comparing apixaban, at a dose of 5 mg twice daily, with placebo, in addition to standard antiplatelet therapy, in patients with a recent acute coronary syndrome and at least two 6._____ (add) risk factors for recurrent ischemic events.

Results

The trial was terminated prematurely after 7._____ (recruit) of 7392 patients because of an increase in major bleeding events with apixaban in the absence of a counter-balancing reduction in recurrent ischemic events. With a median follow-up of 241 days, the primary outcome of cardiovascular death, myocardial infarction, or ischemic stroke occurred in 279 of the 3705 patients (7.5%) 8._____ (assign) to apixaban (13.2 events per 100 patient-years) and in 293 of the 3687 patients (7.9%) 9._____ (assign) to placebo (14.0 events per 100 patient-years) (hazard ratio with apixaban, 0.95; 95% confidence interval [CI], 0.80 to 1.11; P = 0.51). The primary safety outcome of major bleeding according to the Thrombolysis in Myocardial Infarction (TIMI) definition 10._____ (occur) in 46 of the 3673 patients (1.3%) who received at least one dose of apixaban (2.4 events per 100 patient-years) and in 18 of the 3642 patients (0.5%) who received at least one dose of placebo (0.9 events per 100 patient-years) (hazard ratio with apixaban, 2.59; 95% CI, 1.50 to 4.46; P = 0.001). A greater number of intracranial and fatal bleeding events occurred with apixaban than with placebo.

Conclusions

The 11._____ (add) of apixaban, at a dose of 5 mg twice daily, to antiplatelet therapy in highrisk patients after an acute coronary syndrome increased the number of major bleeding events without a significant 12._____ (reduce) in recurrent ischemic events.

3. 阅读下面的句子并重新排序，使之成为一段合理的摘要，并为其撰写合适的标题。

（a）We adapted 10x Visium spatial transcriptomics to determine the identity and in situ location of intratumoral microbial communities within patient tissues.

（b）We developed a single-cell RNA-sequencing method that we name INVADEseq（invasion-adhesion-directed expression sequencing）and，by applying this to patient tumours，identify cell-associated bacteria and the host cells with which they interact，as well as uncovering alterations in transcriptional pathways that are involved in inflammation，metastasis，cell dormancy and DNA repair.

（c）The tumour-associated microbiota is an intrinsic component of the tumour microenvironment across human cancer types.

（d）Here，by applying in situ spatial-profiling technologies and single-cell RNA sequencing to oral squamous cell carcinoma and colorectal cancer，we reveal spatial，cellular and molecular host-microbe interactions.

（e）Using GeoMx digital spatial profiling，we show that bacterial communities populate microniches that are less vascularized，highly immunosuppressive and associated with malignant cells with lower levels of Ki-67 as compared to bacteria-negative tumour regions.

（f）Intratumoral host-microbiota studies have so far largely relied on bulk tissue analysis，which obscures the spatial distribution and localized effect of the microbiota within tumours.

（g）Collectively，our data reveal that the distribution of the microbiota within a tumour is not random；instead，it is highly organized in microniches with immune and epithelial cell functions that promote cancer progression.

（h）Through functional studies，we show that cancer cells that are infected with bacteria invade their surrounding environment as single cells and recruit myeloid cells to bacterial regions.

4. 翻译下列摘要中的句子。

（1）在住院患者中，与安慰剂相比，单次大剂量维生素 D_3 并没有显著缩短住院时间。

_____

_____

（2）在这篇综述中，我们建议补充维生素 D，通过调节成人和儿童人群对病毒的免疫反应，在预防和/或治疗 SARS-CoV-2 感染疾病中发挥作用。

_____

_____

（3）母体妊娠感染是后代发展精神障碍的一个典型危险因素，包括精神分裂症、自闭症和注意力缺陷障碍。感染引起的炎症反应部分是针对胎盘和胎儿的，是胎儿大脑发育异常的假定致病机制。

_____

（4）这是一项多中心、双盲、随机、安慰剂对照试验，在巴西圣保罗的两个地点进行。该研究包括 240 名在 2020 年 6 月 2 日至 2020 年 8 月 27 日入院时病情中度至重度的住院患者。最后一次随访是在 2020 年 10 月 7 日。

_____

第四章 前 言

第一节 前言的功能及主要内容

前言(Introduction),也称引言(Foreword)、导言或序言(Preface),处于论文正文开始位置,为读者简要介绍本研究的背景资料和研究目的。前言是正文的引子,能够起到提纲挈领的作用,激发读者的阅读兴趣,引导读者进入论文的主题。

不同国际期刊在"作者须知"(Instructions for Authors)中都明确了前言部分的写作要求,例如 Science 在"稿件的格式和类型"(Format and style of main manuscript)中对"前言"的要求是:"The manuscript should start with a brief introduction describing the paper's significance. The introduction should provide sufficient background information to make the article intelligible to readers in other disciplines and sufficient context so that the significance of the experimental findings is clear."由此可见,前言的基本功能是提供简洁、易懂的资料阐述研究的内容和目的,让来自不同领域的读者能够明白研究的意义所在,引导读者进一步阅读全文。

一般来说,前言应包括以下主要内容:

(1) 研究的背景资料或研究现状综述(research background or review of research status);

(2) 对前人研究的评论或发现新的研究问题(research problem or research gap);

(3) 本文研究目的或研究假设(research objective or hypothesis);

有的论著在前言部分也可简要概述一下本研究的起始时间、方法、结果及意义。

第二节 前言例文分析

下面,我们具体分析几篇著名国际期刊刊登的学术论文的前言部分。

例 1:

Out-of-hospital cardiac arrest is a common and lethal problem, leading to an estimated 330,000 deaths each year in the United States and Canada. Overall, the rate of survival to hospital discharge among patients with an out-of-hospital cardiac arrest who are treated by emergency medical services (EMS) personnel is low but varies greatly, with rates ranging from 3.0% to 16.3%. This variation in the rate of survival can be attributed partly to local variations in the five key links in the chain of survival: rapid EMS access, early cardiopulmonary resuscitation (CPR), early defibrillation, early advanced cardiac life support, and effective care after resuscitation. Concerted efforts by EMS personnel to strengthen these links have led to only a slight increase in survival rates in recent years.

The traditional approach to out-of-hospital cardiac arrest has been to emphasize early analysis of cardiac rhythm, with delivery of defibrillatory shocks, if indicated, as quickly as possible. It has been suggested, however, that many patients may benefit from a period of CPR before the first analysis of rhythm. The 2005 resuscitation guidelines from the American Heart Association-International Liaison Committee on Resuscitation (AHA-ILCOR) departed from its previous "shock first" strategy by suggesting that responders could provide 2 minutes of CPR before analysis of cardiac rhythm. These changes in the guidelines are supported by the findings of three clinical studies but are not supported by two others, and in the 2010 guidelines, the recommendation was modified to say that "there is inconsistent evidence to support or refute" such a delay in the analysis of cardiac rhythm. Therefore, the preferred initial approach remains uncertain. Our objective was to compare two approaches to the timing of CPR by EMS personnel—a brief period of manual chest compressions and ventilations with prompt initiation of rhythm analysis and defibrillation (early analysis) versus a longer period of compressions and ventilations before the first analysis of cardiac rhythm (later analysis).

[Excerpted from Early versus Later Rhythm Analysis in Patients with Out-of-Hospital Cardiac Arrest. *N Engl J Med.*, 2011, 365(9): 787 - 97.]

【分析】

这是《新英格兰医学杂志》上刊登的一篇学术论文的前言部分,共有 2 个自然段。第 1 自然段主要介绍研究背景,指出院外心搏骤停现象(out-of-hospital cardiac arrest)及影响生存率(the rate of survival)的因素。第 1 自然段共有 4 句,第 1 句首先介绍院外心搏骤停现象造成的危害,第 2 句提出关键词"生存率"及差异性,第 3 句分析造成生存率差异性的主要因素,第 4 句指出当前医疗实践的效果不太明显,由此引起读者对该研究问题的思考。

第 2 自然段针对第 1 自然段提出的研究问题展开进一步论述,该段共有 6 句。其中第 1、2 两句指出传统的抢救方法和引起的争议,随后第 3、4、5 句通过介绍 2 份心脏复苏指南(resuscitation guidelines)的差别,进一步指出当前研究的缺陷及可以研究的方向,也由此为下面介绍本论文研究做了铺垫。最后一句指出本研究的目的,以验证以上分析。

这篇论文的引言从研究背景的概述过渡到对所发现问题的解决设想,呈现"漏斗型"的逻辑框架,即从概述一般研究问题(general topic)到发现特定研究问题(specific topic)到寻求解决特定问题(how to solve it),这种写作思路使读者能够获得较为清晰的研究框架,快速了解研究主题,是学术论文前言常用的写作方法。

【实用短语】

- out-of-hospital cardiac arrest 院外心搏骤停
- the rate of survival 生存率
- emergency medical services 急诊医疗服务
- early cardiopulmonary resuscitation 早期心肺复苏
- concerted efforts 齐心协力
- a slight increase 略微增长
- defibrillatory shocks 除颤电击
- the preferred initial approach 首选的最初方法
- departed from 偏离
- inconsistent evidence 不一致的证据
- cardiac rhythm 心律

【句型模仿】

1. Out-of-hospital cardiac arrest is a common and lethal problem, leading to an estimated 330,000 deaths each year in the United States and Canada.

本句表达"……是一种常见的致命疾病,每年造成约……人死亡",注意现在分词的使用。

2. This variation in the rate of survival can be attributed partly to local variations …

本句中 "can be attributed partly to"意为"可以部分归因于……",注意 to 是介词,后面需跟名词或动名词短语。

【长难句理解】

Overall, the rate of survival to hospital discharge among patients with an out-of-hospital cardiac arrest who are treated by emergency medical services(EMS) personnel is low but varies greatly, with rates ranging from 3.0% to 16.3%.

总体而言,经急诊人员抢救(EMS)的院外心搏骤停患者出院存活率低但差异性较大,存活率从 3% 到 16.3% 不等。

例 2:

Several recent expert summaries have highlighted the health impacts of chronic obstructive pulmonary disease(COPD). In Australia, there were 4761 deaths(4% of all deaths)attributed to COPD in 2006, and 47 207 life were lost due to COPD in

2003. In 2006 - 07, there were 52 560 hospital separations in Australia attributed to COPD, with an average length of stay of 7 days. COPD has a substantial impact on mortality and health service use.

Data on the prevalence of COPD and related symptoms are limited, with estimates ranging from 1.4% to 6.9%, depending on the age group studied and the definitions used. COPD is usually not diagnosed until it is moderately advanced and begins to impair quality of life. Furthermore, due to poor utilisation of spirometry in primary care settings and the largely silent nature of the disease in its early stages, COPD is under-recognised by doctors and underreported by patients. Surveys that have used objective measurement of lung function to identify COPD have found a high proportion of previously undiagnosed cases.

Valid estimation of the prevalence of COPD requires a comprehensive, nationwide, population-based survey, including high-quality post-bronchodilator spirometry, conducted in a representative sample of the population. In collaboration with the international Burden of Obstructive Lung Disease (BOLD) study, we conducted this research to describe the prevalence of obstructive lung disease, including symptoms, diagnoses and level of airflow obstruction, in people aged 40 years or older in Australia.

[Excerpted from Respiratory symptoms and illness in older Australians: the Burden of Obstructive Lung Disease (BOLD) study. *The Medical Journal of Australia*, 2013, 198(3): 144 - 148.]

【分析】

这是一篇澳大利亚有关慢性阻塞性肺病(chronic obstructive pulmonary disease, COPD)学术论文的前言部分。该前言共分 3 个自然段,第 1 自然段主要介绍背景,描述慢性阻塞性肺病在澳大利亚的发病情况和造成的影响。第 2 自然段聚焦 COPD 的一个特征,即前期症状不明显,及检测设备的不足造成 COPD 早期诊断的困难。第 3 自然段在前 2 段的基础上,介绍了本研究的内容,即在澳大利亚 40 周岁以上人群中展开慢性阻塞性肺病发病率的研究,包括症状、诊断及气流阻塞程度等内容。

这段前言的写作逻辑非常清晰,从描述一般情况(general condition)到聚焦研究中的某一点(specific condition),由此顺理成章地指出本文研究重点及意义所在,是一篇很好的范文。

【实用短语】

• an average length of stay 平均住院时长

• related symptoms 相关症状

• have a substantial impact on 有明显的影响

• moderately advanced 中度晚期

- impair quality of life 降低生活质量
- primary care settings 初级保健机构
- silent nature of the disease in its early stages 疾病早期症状不明显
- a high proportion of 相当比例的
- previously undiagnosed cases 以前未确诊的病例
- a representative sample of the population 代表性的人口样本
- in collaboration with 与……合作
- conduct this research 开展本研究
- people aged 40 years or older 40 岁及以上人群

【句型模仿】

1. Several recent expert summaries <u>have highlighted the health impacts of</u> chronic obstructive pulmonary disease (COPD).

本句中的"highlight the health impacts of"意为"强调……的健康影响"。

2. In 2006 - 07, <u>there were 52 560 hospital separations</u> in Australia <u>attributed to</u> COPD, <u>with an average length of stay of 7 days.</u>

本句画线部分描述"由于……疾病导致住院人数为……，平均住院时长为……天"。

3. <u>Data on the prevalence of</u> COPD and related symptoms <u>are limited</u>, <u>with estimates ranging</u> from 1.4% to 6.9%, <u>depending on</u> the age group studied and the definitions used.

本句介绍 COPD 现行研究的数据不足和患病率的估测范围，借助 with 短语和分词短语"depending on"构成复合句，将原本松散的短句合成一个结构紧凑、意义完整的句子，这也是中英文语言的主要区别之一。

【长难句理解】

1. Furthermore, due to poor utilisation of spirometry in primary care settings and the largely silent nature of the disease in its early stages, COPD is under-recognised by doctors and underreported by patients.

此外，由于初级保健机构对肺活量测定利用率不足，以及该疾病在早期阶段症状不明显，COPD 没有得到医生的充分认识，患者的报告也较少。

2. Surveys that have used objective measurement of lung function to identify COPD have found a high proportion of previously undiagnosed cases.

使用肺功能客观测量来识别 COPD 的调查发现，以前未确诊的病例比例很高。

3. Valid estimation of the prevalence of COPD requires a comprehensive, nationwide, population-based survey, including high-quality post-bronchodilator spirometry, conducted in a representative sample of the population.

有效评估 COPD 的患病率需要在全国范围内进行全面的、基于人群的调查，包括在具有代表性的人口样本中进行高质量的支气管扩张剂后肺活量测定。

第三节 前言的语言特征与常用句型

3.1 前言部分时态的运用

前言部分动词时态依据表述内容来定。下面进行详细分析。

（1）在介绍研究的背景、现状和尚未解决的问题时，常用一般现在时和现在完成时。

例1：Asthma and hypertension <u>are</u> common chronic diseases, each with attendant morbidity, mortality, and economic effects. <u>It is estimated</u> that 300 million people worldwide <u>have</u> asthma, and an increase in prevalence to 400 million <u>is anticipated by</u> 2025.

哮喘和高血压是常见慢性病，每种疾病都伴随着发病率、死亡率和经济影响。据估计，全世界有3亿人患有哮喘，预计到2025年患病者将增至4亿。

例2：Worldwide estimates <u>suggest</u> that 874 million adults have a systolic blood pressure higher than 140 mm Hg, and the prevalence of hypertension, like that of asthma, <u>is</u> increasing, along with costs, morbidity, and mortality.

据估计，全球有8.74亿成年人的收缩压高于140毫米汞柱，像哮喘一样，高血压的治疗费用、发病率和死亡率都在增加。

（2）描述研究过程中的主要活动，包括资料的来源和收集、研究的起始时间和主要方法时，常用一般过去时和过去完成时。

例3：The VADT follow-up study（VADT-F）<u>was designed to</u> examine long-term consequences of intensive glycemic control on cardiovascular disease outcomes, quality of life, and mortality and, as previously reported, provides an opportunity for assessing legacy effects.

VADT随访研究（VADT-F）旨在检查强化血糖控制对心血管疾病结局、生活质量和死亡率的长期影响，如前所述，它为评估遗留效应提供了机会。

例4：We <u>conducted</u> an investigator-led, randomized clinical trial, ADVANCE, to evaluate the efficacy and safety of two antiretroviral therapy（ART）combinations, TAF-FTC-DTG and TDF-FTC-DTG, as compared with the current first-line regimen of TDF-FTC（or 3TC）-EFV used in the majority of patients in low- and middle-income countries.

注：tenofovir alafenamide fumarate（TAF） tenofovir disoproxil fumarate（TDF） dolutegravir（DTG） lamivudine（3TC） emtricitabine（FTC） efavirenz（EFV）

我们开展了一项由研究者主导的随机临床试验 ADVEST，以评估两种抗反转录病毒疗法（ART）组合，即 TAF-FTC-DTG 和 TDF-FTC-DTG 的疗效和安全性，并与目前用于中低收入国家大多数患者的一线治疗方案 TDF-FTC（或 3TC）-EFV 进行比较。

（3）说明本研究的内容时，常用一般过去时。在说明本文的写作目的时，常用一般现在时。这点与摘要中"目的"部分的写作要求相同。

例 5：Our trial <u>evaluated</u> the 1-year efficacy of refillable e-cigarettes as compared with nicotine replacement when provided to adults seeking help to quit smoking and combined with face-to-face behavioral support.

当给寻求戒烟的成年人提供帮助，并结合面对面的行为支持时，我们的试验评估了与尼古丁替代物相比，持续使用 1 年可再填充电子烟的疗效。

例 6：In this review, we <u>discuss</u> the potential mechanistic links between hypertension and asthma, the influence each condition has on the other, and approaches to the treatment of hypertension in adult patients with asthma.

这篇综述讨论了高血压和哮喘之间的潜在机制联系，两种疾病的相互影响，以及成年哮喘患者高血压的治疗方法。

3.2　前言部分常用的句型

医学论文的前言部分需要提供一定的背景资料，并对自己的研究进行概述，其中涉及的常用英文表达形式有很多。下面将经常出现的句型和表达方式分类总结，以方便大家模仿和使用。

3.2.1　表达背景材料时

【常用句型】

- It has been reported/demonstrated/observed that ... 据报道/证实/观察……

- ... are well documented 关于……有充分的记录

- Over the course of the past 20 years,... has emerged 在过去的 20 年里，……已经出现

- Several lines of evidence suggest that ... 多项证据表明……

- Previous studies have demonstrated/indicated/shown that ... 以往的研究表明（显示）……

- Several recent expert summaries have highlighted ... 近来几篇专家摘要都强调了……

例 7：In patients with diabetic kidney disease with increased levels of albuminuria, <u>large placebo-controlled trials have shown</u> that renin-angiotensin system（RAS）inhibitors, sodium-glucose cotransporter 2（SGLT2）inhibitors, and the non-steroidal mineralocorticoid receptor antagonist finerenone all reduced the risk of progression to kidney failure.

在蛋白尿水平升高的糖尿病肾病患者中,大型安慰剂对照试验表明,肾素-血管紧张素系统(RAS)抑制剂、钠-葡萄糖协同转运蛋白 2(SGLT2)抑制剂和非甾体矿物皮质激素受体拮抗剂 finerenone 均可降低进展为肾衰竭的风险。

例 8:Horizontal transmission of bacteria, especially multidrug-resistant organisms (MDROs), <u>remains an important concern in hospitals worldwide.</u>

细菌的水平传播,尤其是耐多药生物的水平传播,仍然是全世界医院关注的一个重要问题。

例 9:The adverse health effects of short-term exposure to ambient air pollution <u>are well documented.</u> Particulate matter(PM), especially, arouses public health concerns because of its toxicity and the widespread human exposure to this pollutant.

短期暴露于环境空气污染对健康的不利影响已有充分的记录。特别是颗粒物,由于其毒性和人类广泛接触这种污染物,引起了公共卫生关注。

3.2.2 表达发现的问题或以往研究的不足时

【常用句型】

• Little research has been done about … 关于……研究做得很少

• … remains controversial/unexplored/unclear/elusive/uncertain 关于……的研究仍有争议,尚不清楚

• There are still questions/debates/conflicting results about … 仍然存在有关……的问题/争论/矛盾的结论

• However, only limited data are available with regard to … 然而,有关……的数据仍然有限

• The mechanisms underlying … are unknown. 有关……的机制尚不清楚。

• Although a lot of effort is being spent on …, the efficient and effective methods has yet to be developed. 虽然人们在……方面做了大量努力,但有效的方法还有待研究。

例 10:<u>There are questions about</u> risks and benefits of use of e-cigarettes for different purposes, but an important clinical issue is whether e-cigarette use in a quit attempt facilitates success, particularly as compared with the use of nicotine-replacement therapy.

人们对出于不同目的使用电子烟的风险和益处存在疑问,但有一个重要的临床问题是,所有的戒烟尝试中使用电子烟是否有助于成功戒烟,特别是与使用尼古丁替代疗法相比。

例 11:<u>Although</u> overall obesity <u>has been clearly associated with</u> an increased risk of death, the association of overweight (BMI, 25.0 to 29.9) with risk of death has been inconsistent.

尽管全身肥胖与死亡风险增加明显相关,但超重(BMI,25.0—29.9)与死亡风险之间的关联一直不一致。

3.2.3 表达本研究的目的或意义时

【常用句型】

- In the present study, we aim to ... 在当前研究中,我们打算……
- The purpose of this study was ... 本研究的目的是……
- Therefore, our first objective in these studies was to determine whether ... 因此,这些研究的首要目的是确定……
- We need to provide more data about ... 我们需要提供更多有关……的数据
- The aim of this paper is to provide ... 本文目的是……
- The present study was undertaken to ... 当前进行的研究是……
- Therefore, ... has practical significance/implication for ... 因此,……对……具有现实意义/启示

例 12：Identifying the features of microbiome transmission will advance our understanding of the complexity of the human microbiome, and can help address the "communicable" factor that microbiome transmission adds to diseases and conditions currently considered non-communicable. Here, we characterize and quantify the patterns of person-to-person microbiome strain sharing across multiple scenarios to provide a comprehensive description of the microbiome transmission landscape.

确定微生物组传播的特征将促进我们对人类微生物组复杂性的理解,并有助于明确那些由微生物组传播引起的疫病及造成疾病传染的条件,这些疾病和条件目前可能被认为不具有传染性。在这里,我们描述和量化多个场景下人际间微生物组菌株共享模式,以提供对微生物组传播情况的全面描述。

例 13：It is important for the clinician to recognize cytokine storm because it has prognostic and therapeutic implications. In this review, we propose a unifying definition of cytokine storm; discuss the pathophysiological features, clinical presentation, and management of the syndrome; and provide an overview of iatrogenic, pathogen-induced, neoplasia-induced, and monogenic causes. Our goal is to provide physicians with a conceptual framework, a unifying definition, and essential staging, assessment, and therapeutic tools to manage cytokine storm.

对于临床医师而言,识别细胞因子风暴非常重要,因为它具有预后和治疗意义。在这篇综述中,我们为细胞因子风暴提出了统一定义;讨论了该综合征的病理生理学特征、临床表现和治疗;并且概述了以下几方面病因:医源性、病原体诱发、肿瘤诱发和单

基因病因。我们的目标是为医师提供概念框架,统一定义,以及控制细胞因子风暴所必需的分期、评估和治疗工具。

第四节　练习巩固

1. 阅读下列医学论文的前言部分,并译成汉语,体会其中的语言特征。

Acute exacerbations of chronic obstructive pulmonary disease (COPD) result in frequent visits to physicians' offices and emergency rooms and numerous hospitalizations and days lost from work; they also account for a substantial percentage of the cost of treating COPD. Patients who have acute exacerbations of COPD, as compared with patients with COPD who do not have acute exacerbations, have an increased risk of death, a more rapid decline in lung function, and reduced quality of life. Although inhaled glucocorticoids, long-acting beta 2-agonists, and long-acting muscarinic antagonists reduce the frequency of acute exacerbations of COPD, patients receiving all three of these medications may still have as many as 1.4 acute exacerbations, on average, each year.

Macrolide antibiotics have immunomodulatory, antiinflammatory, and antibacterial effects. Seven small studies that tested whether macrolides decrease the frequency of acute exacerbations of COPD reported conflicting results. Accordingly, we conducted a large, randomized trial to test the hypothesis that zithromycin decreases the frequency of acute exacerbations of COPD when added to the usual care of these patients.

2. 请将下列前言部分的句子翻译成英语。

(1) 以锻炼为基础的心脏康复是对稳定型心绞痛(chronic stable angina)和心肌梗死(MI)或接受过冠状动脉旁路移植术手术(coronary artery bypass grafting,CABG)病人的长效管理机制的一个重要组成部分。

_____

_____

(2) 据报道,对冠心病患者来说,相比不参与心脏康复而言,参与心脏康复是有益的。

_____

_____

(3) 对医疗保险受益人的分析也发现,在因冠心病住院的患者中,存在与参与心脏康复相关联的生存获益(survival benefit)。

_____

_____

（4）在参与心脏康复的患者中，关于最佳心脏康复"剂量"的证据是有限的。

（5）在本研究中，针对一群参与心脏康复的医疗保险受益人，我们试图描述参加心脏康复时间与心肌梗死之间的剂量—反应关系。

3. 以下是两篇学术论文的前言部分，但顺序排列错误，请将句子重新排序，并分析每个句子的功能。

Article 1

A. Although transmission of ZIKV has declined in the Americas, outbreaks and infection clusters continue to occur in some regions, such as India and South-east Asia, where there are large populations of women of childbearing age who are susceptible to the virus.

B. The ability of ZIKV to cause congenital defects in fetuses and infants, as exemplified by the microcephaly epidemic in Brazil, is an unprecedented feature in a mosquito-borne viral infection.

C. We review the body of information that was acquired during the pandemic and discuss the epidemiologic trends, current knowledge about the transmission and natural history of ZIKV infection and its sequelae, and the principles of diagnosis and clinical management.

D. Zika virus (ZIKV) was discovered in Africa in 1947 and was first detected in Asia in 1966, yet its potential effect on public health was not recognized until the virus caused outbreaks in the Pacific from 2007 to 2015 and began spreading throughout the Americas in 2015.

Article 2

A. Yet, the indications for postoperative transfusion have not been adequately evaluated and remain controversial.

B. Blood transfusions are frequently given to surgical patients and to the elderly.

C. Most clinical trials have been small.

D. In the United States, more than 17 million red-cell units are collected annually, and 15 million units are transfused.

E. We performed the Transfusion Trigger Trial for Functional Outcomes in Cardiovascular Patients Undergoing Surgical Hip Fracture Repair (FOCUS) to test the hypothesis that a higher threshold for blood transfusion (a hemoglobin level of

10 g per deciliter) would improve functional recovery and reduce morbidity and mortality, as compared with a more restrictive transfusion strategy (a hemoglobin level of <8 g per deciliter or symptoms).

F. However, the effect of a restrictive approach on functional recovery or risk of myocardial infarction in patients with cardiac disease has not been studied.

G. One adequately powered trial involving adults in intensive care units showed a nonsignificant decrease in 30-day mortality with a restrictive transfusion strategy, as compared with a liberal strategy (18.7% vs. 23.3%).

第五章　研究材料与方法

第一节　研究材料与方法的主要内容

研究材料与方法（Materials and Methods）是学术论文的一个重要组成部分，主要向读者说明通过哪些技术途径、采用何种研究方法、如何解决研究问题以及数据统计分析的处理方法等等，其主要功能有二：一是为读者了解研究成果的可靠性和可信性提供依据，二是为其他研究者以后开展类似研究时提供参考和借鉴。因此，作者必须对研究的材料和方法进行全面详尽的介绍，为论文结果的科学性提供基础和依据。

很多国际医学学术期刊会在"作者须知"（Instructions for Authors）中说明这一部分的写作要求。"材料"应包括研究对象、性质、来源、数量、所使用仪器、设备、装置等内容，"方法"应包括研究设计、分组情况、数据统计、误差分析等内容。在写作过程中，通常会以小标题（subtitle）来呈现各部分详细内容。一般来说，材料与方法的主要内容包括以下四个方面：

- 研究设计（study design）
- 研究对象（study subjects）
- 研究方法（study method）
- 统计分析（statistical analysis）

同时，在进行这部分写作时，还需注意以下几个方面：

（1）提供足够多的细节，读者无须回顾以往的文献就可了解采用的具体方法。

（2）详细说明研究对象，包括患者、实验动物、组织、细胞以及生物分子材料等。例如患者要说明人数、性别、年龄、健康状况、疾病状况等，动物则要说明种系、等级、数量、来源、性别、年龄、体重、饲养条件和健康状况等，而细胞则要说明来源、类别、产地及培养条件等等，还需提供伦理委员会的批准证明或患者的知情同意书。

（3）实验中的仪器、设备等，一定要交代清楚型号、规格、生产单位等细节，药品试剂要使用化学名称，注明剂量、批号、单位、纯度、生产单位等。

（4）统计学分析是材料与方法中不可缺少的一项，也是重要的一项内容。注意在这个小标题下交代清楚所使用的统计学方法、数据的表示方法等内容即可，不必过多介绍统计分析工具和结果，因为那是留待在论文"结果"部分详述的。

（5）在英语时态选择上,这一部分大都采用过去时或过去完成时,以描述研究实施过程和所采用的方法。

第二节 研究材料与方法例文分析

下面,举例分析学术论文的"材料与方法"写作部分。

例:**Methods**

Study Oversight

The executive steering committee designed and oversaw the conduct of the trial and data analysis in collaboration with representatives of the study sponsor (Pfizer). The trial was monitored by an independent data and safety monitoring committee. Data were collected, managed, and analyzed by the sponsor according to a predefined statistical analysis plan, and the analyses were replicated by an independent academic statistician. The manuscript was prepared by an academic writing group, whose members had unrestricted access to the data, and was subsequently revised by all the authors. All the authors made the decision to submit the manuscript for publication and assume responsibility for the accuracy and completeness of the data and analyses.

Study Patients

The design of the EMPHASIS-HF trial has been published in detail, and the trial protocol and statistical analysis plan are available at NEJM. org. The trial was approved by each center's ethics committee. All patients provided written informed consent.

Eligibility criteria were as follows: an age of at least 55 years, NYHA functional class Ⅱ symptoms, an ejection fraction of no more than 30% (or, if >30 to 35%, a QRS duration of > 130 m sec on electrocardiography), and treatment with an angiotensin-converting-enzyme (ACE) inhibitor, an angiotensin-receptor blocker (ARB), or both and a beta-blocker (unlesscontraindicated) at the recommended dose or maximal tolerated dose.

Randomization was to occur within 6 months after hospitalization for a cardiovascular reason. Patients who had not been hospitalized for a cardiovascular reason within 6 months before the screening visit could be enrolled if the plasma level of B-type natriuretic peptide (BNP) was at least 250 pg per milliliter or if the plasma level of N-terminal pro-BNP was at least 500 pg per milliliter in men and 750 pg per milliliter in women.

Key exclusion criteria were acute myocardial infarction, NYHA class Ⅲ or Ⅳ heart failure, a serum potassium level exceeding 5.0 mmol per liter, an estimated glomerular filtration rate (GFR) of less than 30 ml per minute per 1.73 m² of body-surface area, a need for a potassium-sparing diuretic, and any other clinically significant, coexisting condition.

Study Procedures

We used a computerized randomization system involving concealed study-group assignments to randomly assign patients to receive eplerenone or matching placebo. Eplerenone was started at a dose of 25 mg once daily and was increased after 4 weeks to 50 mg once daily (or started at 25 mg on alternate days, and increased to 25 mg daily, if the estimated GFR was 30 to 49 ml per minute per 1.73 m2), provided the serum potassium level was no more than 5.0 mmol per liter.

Thereafter, investigators evaluated patients every 4 months and were instructed to decrease the dose of the study drug if the serum potassium level was 5.5 to 5.9 mmol per liter and to withhold the study drug if the serum potassium level was 6.0 mmol per liter or more. Potassium was to be remeasured within 72 hours after the dose reduction or study-drug withdrawal, and the study drug was to be restarted only if the level was below 5.0 mmol per liter.

Study Outcomes

The primary outcome was a composite of death from cardiovascular causes or a first hospitalization for heart failure. The prespecified adjudicated secondary outcomes were hospitalization for heart failure or death from any cause, death from any cause, death from cardiovascular causes, hospitalization for any reason, and hospitalization for heart failure, among others. Adjudication of the outcomes was carried out by an independent committee according to prespecified criteria.

Statistical Analysis

The initial assumptions were that, with 2 584 patients and an annual event rate of 18% in the placebo group (based on data from a subgroup analysis of the Candesartan in Heart Failure: Assessment of Reduction in Mortality and Morbidity-Added Trial), our trial would require 813 patients with a primary outcome occurring within 48 months to achieve 80% power to detect an 18% relative reduction in the risk of the primary outcome in the eplerenone group as compared with the placebo group (with a two-sided alpha of 0.05). Because the overall blinded event rate was lower than expected, the sample size was increased to 3 100 patients, according to a protocol amendment adopted in June 2009.

The data and safety monitoring committee's charter specified interim analyses of the primary outcome after approximately 271 and 542 events had occurred, with a statistical stopping guideline for an overwhelming benefit (two-sided $P < 0.001$ in favor of eplerenone). On May 6, 2010, after the second interim analysis, the data and safety monitoring committee reported to the executive committee chairs that the prespecified stopping boundary for an overwhelming benefit had been crossed. The full executive committee was informed, decided to stop the trial, and notified the sponsor of this decision on May 9, 2010. Operationally, May 25, 2010, was chosen as the trial cutoff date for all efficacy and safety analyses reported here.

Comparability of baseline characteristics between the two study groups was assessed by means of a two-sample t-test, for continuous variables, or Fisher's exact test, for categorical variables. The analyses of the adjudicated primary and secondary outcomes were conducted on data from all patients who had undergone randomization, according to the intention-to-treat principle, with the use of Kaplan-Meier estimates and Cox proportional-hazards models. Hazard ratios, 95% confidence intervals, and P values were calculated with the use of models adjusted for the following prespecified baseline prognostic factors: age, estimated GFR, ejection fraction, body-mass index, hemoglobin value, heart rate, systolic blood pressure, diabetes mellitus, history of hypertension, previous myocardial infarction, atrial fibrillation, and left bundle-branch block or QRS duration greater than 130 m sec. Sensitivity analyses were also performed, by means of unadjusted Cox models.

The consistency of the treatment effect was assessed among 20 prespecified subgroups. The effect in each subgroup was analyzed with the use of a Cox proportional-hazards model, without adjustment for covariates. The treatment-by-subgroup interaction was evaluated by means of a Cox proportional-hazards model with terms for treatment, subgroup, and their interaction.

The number of patients who would need to be treated to prevent one primary-outcome event from occurring was determined according to the method of Altman and Andersen. Post hoc comparisons between the two groups of the total number of hospitalizations for any reason and for heart failure were performed with the use of a t-test, assuming a Poisson distribution. Serious adverse events, anticipated adverse events, and adverse events leading to permanent study-drug withdrawal were tabulated according to randomized group assignment and analyzed by means of Fisher's exact test.

[Excerpted from Eplerenone in Patients with Systolic Heart Failure and Mild Symptoms. *N Engl J Med*, 2011, 364(1): 11-21.]

【分析】

这是一篇关于收缩期心衰和有轻度症状的病人使用强心剂(Eplerenone,中文名依普利酮)的论文。该论文的方法部分分为几个小标题:Study Oversight(研究监管)、Study Patients(研究对象)、Study Procedures(研究过程)、Study Outcomes(研究结果)

和 Statistical Analysis(研究分析)。在 Study Oversight 部分中,作者交代了本研究学术监管委员会与赞助商及每个机构的具体职责。在 Study Patients 部分中,作者首先说明该研究得到了伦理委员会的批准,并且患者本人也签署了知情同意书,然后详细说明研究对象的入选标准和排除标准。在 Study Procedures 部分中,作者交代了研究方法,包括随机分组、药品剂量及用法等。在 Study Outcomes 部分中,作者依次说明主要转归和次要转归的主要情况。而在最后一部分 Statistical Analysis 中,作者交代得比较详细,首先说明数据的来源,然后描述采用何种分析方法。

【实用短语】

• design and oversee the conduct of the trial and data analysis 设计、监管实验的进行和数据的分析

• have unrestricted access to the data 不受限制访问数据

• submit the manuscript for publication 投稿以期发表

• assume responsibility for the accuracy and completeness of the data and analyses 为数据和分析的准确性、完整性负责

• written informed consent 书面知情同意书

• eligibility criteria 入选标准

• exclusion criteria 排除标准

• at the recommended dose 按照建议剂量

• maximal tolerated dose 最大耐受剂量

• acute myocardial infarction 急性心肌梗死

• glomerular filtration rate (GFR) 肾小球滤过率

• potassium-sparing diuretic 保钾利尿剂

• computerized randomization system 机辅随机分组系统

• on alternate days 隔天进行

• withhold the study drug 终止试验药物

• primary outcome 主要转归

• secondary outcome 次要转归

【句型模仿】

1. The executive steering committee designed and oversaw the conduct of the trial and data analysis in collaboration with representatives of the study sponsor (Pfizer).

本句描述"与……合作,共同设计、监管该实验的进行和数据分析",注意动词"design"和"oversee"的并列使用,介词短语"in collaboration with"引导该句的状语成分,使得本句结构紧凑。

2. Data were collected, managed, and analyzed by the sponsor according to a predefined statistical analysis plan, and the analyses were replicated by an

independent academic statistician.

本句两处画线部分同为被动语态的并列结构，这在学术论方法部分中是常见的，隐去施动者，描述行为本身，凸显客观、实事求是的态度。"Data were collected, managed, and analyzed by"意为"数据由……进行收集、处理和分析"，"were replicated by"意为"由……复制"。

3. Randomization was to occur within 6 months after hospitalization for a cardiovascular reason.

本句仍然使用被动语态描述实验方法。当句子无须交代动作的发出者，读者也会明白是谁开展了这个实验，或是当突出动作的实施对象时，被动语态通常比主动语态更加客观、直接。本句使用"randomization（随机分配）"作主语，突出采取的分组方法。本句另请注意介词"for"的用法，"be hospitalized for"或"hospitalization for"表示"因为……而住院"。

4. We used a computerized randomization system involving concealed study-group assignments to randomly assign patients to receive eplerenone or matching placebo.

本句分别出现了"assign"的名词形式"assignments"和动词形式"assign"，前者在词组"concealed study-group assignments"中表示"隐匿的研究分组任务"，后者出现在词组"randomly assign ... to ... "中，表示"随机分配"，是方法中表示分组方法的常用短语。

5. The primary outcome was a composite of death from cardiovascular causes or a first hospitalization for heart failure.

本句中"outcome"意为"疾病的转归"，"a composite of death from"表示"由于……导致的合并死亡"，"a first hospitalization for"表示"由于……导致的首次住院"。

【长难句理解】

1. Patients who had not been hospitalized for a cardiovascular reason within 6 months before the screening visit could be enrolled if the plasma level of B-type natriuretic peptide (BNP) was at least 250 pg per milliliter or if the plasma level of N-terminal pro-BNP was at least 500 pg per milliliter in men and 750 pg per milliliter in women.

患者在筛查前 6 个月内未因心血管原因住院，如果 B 型利钠肽（BNP）血浆水平至少 250 pg/ml，或血浆的 N 端前 BNP 水平男性至少为 500 pg/ml，女性至少为 750 pg/ml，则可纳入研究。

2. Potassium was to be remeasured within 72 hours after the dose reduction or study-drug withdrawal, and the study drug was to be restarted only if the level was below 5.0 mmol per liter.

在减少剂量或停用研究药物后 72 小时内重新测量钾含量，且只有当研究药物的水平低于每升 5.0 mmol 时才重新开始使用。

3. Serious adverse events, anticipated adverse events, and adverse events leading

to permanent study-drug withdrawal were tabulated according to randomized group assignment and analyzed by means of Fisher's exact test.

根据随机分组,将严重不良事件、预期不良事件和导致永久停药的不良事件制成表格,并采用 Fisher 精确检验进行分析。

第三节　研究材料与方法的语言特征与常用句型

"材料与方法"作为医学学术论文的一项重要组成部分,在英文表达上有其特殊的时态运用和一些常见的表达句型。下面逐一进行分析。

3.1　材料与方法部分时态的运用

"材料与方法"部分是对研究过程的回顾性描述,动词常用一般过去时。

例 1:To ensure we covered a broad range of the available literature, we searched the reference lists of relevant studies, websites of pertinent professional bodies (eg, FDA), non-governmental organizations, and grey literature (eg, reports or conference abstracts), and we contacted experts in the field to recommend relevant reports.

为确保我们涵盖了广泛的可用文献,我们搜索了相关研究的参考文献列表、相关专业机构(如食品和药物管理局)网站、非政府组织网站和灰色文献(如报告或会议摘要),并联系了该领域的专家推荐相关报告。

例 2：We conducted a cross-sectional survey using a self-administered questionnaire to eligible physicians in the United States between May 2018 and August 2018. The questionnaire was voluntary and anonymous, and it was delivered through electronic mail and online forums such as Facebook.

在 2018 年 5 月至 2018 年 8 月期间,我们使用自填式问卷对美国符合条件的医生进行了一项横向调查。问卷是自愿和匿名的,通过电子邮件和脸书等在线论坛发送。

除了一般过去时以外,在材料与方法部分中还会使用过去完成时,以便说明研究或实验某步骤发生之前的动作或情况。请看以下例子:

例 3:Given the pragmatic nature of this trial, the research team was unable to enforce strict adherence to randomization. Accordingly, we modified our protocol to continue the trial until an adequate sample size had been achieved among women receiving the one-step approach and to include additional statistical analyses to account for non-adherence.

鉴于该试验的实用性,研究小组无法严格遵守随机化。因此,我们修改了我们的方案以继续试验,直到接受一步法的女性达到足够的样本量,并纳入额外的统计分析以解释不依从性。

例 4:During home visits, mothers or caregivers were asked whether the child had symptoms of infection (i. e. , diarrhea [defined as at least 3 loose or liquid stools per day], bloody diarrhea, vomiting, fever, or cough or breathing difficulty) and the number of days in the previous week (during the intervention period) or previous 2 weeks (during the follow-up period) that they had occurred.

在家访期间,母亲或护理人员被问及孩子是否有感染症状[即腹泻(每天至少 3 次稀便或液体便)、血性腹泻、呕吐、发烧或咳嗽或呼吸困难],以及在前一周(干预期间)或前两周(随访期间)出现这些症状的天数。

3.2 材料与方法部分的常用句型

材料与方法部分涉及的内容较多,常用的英文表达句型也多种多样。

3.2.1 表达分组的句型

【常用句型】

• ... were randomly allocated to/were randomized into ... 被随机分配到

• ... were divided into/grouped into/classified into/assigned to ... 被分成、分组、分类、分配到

• Randomization was to be taken between ... and ... 在……之间采取分配

例 5:Each of the 10 participating ROC centers (or sites) was divided into approximately 20 subunits, designated as "clusters," according to EMS agency or geographic boundaries or according to defibrillator device, ambulance, station, or battalion. Randomization of clusters was stratified according to site.

根据急救机构、地理边界、除颤设备、救护车、站点或营地等情况,10 个参与的 ROC 中心(或站点)中的每一个被划分为大约 20 个亚单位,这些亚单位被称为"小组群"。随机分组根据地点进行分层。

例 6:Patients in the early-analysis group were assigned to receive 30 to 60 seconds of chest compressions and ventilations (sufficient time to place defibrillator electrodes) before electrocardiographic (ECG) analysis, and those in the late-analysis group were assigned to receive 3 minutes of chest compressions and ventilations before ECG analysis.

早期分析组患者在心电图分析前接受 30—60 秒胸外按压和通气(足够时间放置除颤器电极),晚期分析组患者在心电图分析前接受 3 分钟胸外按压和通气。

3.2.2　表达研究对象入选或淘汰的句型

【常用句型】

- ... were enrolled in/at ...　纳入研究

- ... were considered eligible/ineligible for ...　被认为符合/不符合

- (patients/subjects) entered into the study（患者/研究对象）参加本研究

- Eligibility(Inclusion)/Exclusion criteria were as follows ...　入选/淘汰标准如下

- ... were recruited from ...　选自……

例 7：In this ancillary study, we examined the effects of supplemental vitamin D_3 as compared with placebo on incident fractures in 25,871 U. S. men (age, $\geqslant$50 years) and women (age, $\geqslant$55 years), including 5,106 Black participants, who <u>were enrolled from</u> all 50 states and followed for a median of 5.3 years.

在辅助研究中,我们研究了补充维生素 D_3 与安慰剂对 25 871 名美国男性(年龄$\geqslant$50 岁)和女性(年龄$\geqslant$55 岁)意外骨折的影响(其中包括 5106 名黑人参与者),他们来自所有 50 个州,随访中位时间为 5.3 年。

例 8：We <u>included</u> all persons 18 years of age or older who had an out-of-hospital cardiac arrest that was not the result of trauma and who were treated with defibrillation, delivery of chest compressions, or both by EMS providers.

我们纳入了所有 18 岁或以上的非创伤性院外心脏骤停患者,他们接受了急救医生除颤、胸外按压或两者兼有的治疗。

例 9：We <u>screened</u> children 7.5 to 8.5 months of age. Children with marked anemia (a hemoglobin level of <8.0 g per deciliter), current febrile illness, severe acute malnutrition, a known inherited red-cell disorder or previous transfusion, or known developmental delay were <u>excluded</u>.

我们对 7.5 至 8.5 个月大的儿童进行了筛查,排除了有明显贫血(血红蛋白水平低于 8.0 克/分升)、当前发热、严重急性营养不良、患有遗传性红细胞疾病或既往输血或明显发育迟缓的儿童。

3.2.3　表达诊断或治疗等句型

【常用句型】

- ... was diagnosed as 被诊断为……疾病患者

- ... was diagnosed with/as having ...　被诊断患有……疾病

- Diagnosis of ... was confirmed/established.　确诊患有……疾病

- ... be treated by/with 用……方法治疗

- ... was on ... therapy 接受……方法治疗

- be hospitalized for ... 因为……而住院治疗

例 10：Women <u>received a diagnosis of</u> gestational diabetes if the fasting blood glucose level was at least 92 mg per deciliter (5.1 mmol per liter)，the timed glucose measurement was at least 180 mg per deciliter (10.0 mmol per liter) at 1 hour，or the timed measurement was at least 153 mg per deciliter (8.5 mmol per liter) at 2 hours.

孕妇如果空腹血糖水平至少为 92 毫克/分升(5.1 毫摩尔/升)，1 小时定时血糖测量至少为 180 毫克/分升(10.0 毫摩尔/升)，或 2 小时定时血糖测量至少为 153 毫克/分升(8.5 毫摩尔/升)，则被诊断为患有妊娠期糖尿病。

例 11：The two groups were balanced with respect to baseline characteristics，and all the patients were <u>receiving recommended</u> pharmacologic <u>therapy</u> for systolic heart failure.

两组在基线特征方面是平衡的，所有患者都接受推荐的收缩期心力衰竭药物治疗。

3.2.4　表达倍数、比例、数值的句型

【常用句型】

- ratio of A to B/A：B ratio AB 之比为……
- range from ... to ... /with a range of ... to ... /vary between ... and ... 数值在……之间
- the mean/average age of the control group was ... 对照组的平均年龄为……
- the median time to progression was ... 疾病进展时间中位数为……
- ... episodes of cramp 痉挛次数发作……次
- A is 3 times as long as B/The length of A is 3 times the length of B/A is 3 times longer than B. A 的长度是 B 的三倍。

例 12：The training of participating EMS providers emphasized uninterrupted chest compressions except for required ventilations，with <u>compressions and ventilations</u> applied in a <u>30：2 ratio</u>，and specified that advanced airway devices were to be placed with minimal interruptions to compressions.

医务人员参与的急救培训强调除必要的通气外，还需不间断的胸外按压，按压与通气的比例为 30：2，并规定提前放置气道设备时应尽量减少按压中断。

例 13：<u>All episodes of</u> cardiac arrest in a cluster were randomly assigned to one CPR strategy；after a set period of time，ranging from 3 to 12 months，<u>all episodes</u> in that cluster were then assigned to the other strategy.

一组中所有的心脏骤停被随机分配一种心脏复苏术；一段时间后(3 个月到 12 个月不等)，改用另一种方法。

例 14：This is a validated scale，<u>ranging from</u> 0 to 6，that is commonly used for measuring the performance of daily activities by people who have had a stroke.

这是一个经过验证的量表,范围从 0 到 6,通常用于测量中风患者的日常活动表现。

例 15:Mean scores on the modified Rankin scale <u>were compared between the two treatment groups with the use of</u> a linear model.

采用线性模型比较两个治疗组在改良 Rankin 量表上的平均得分。

3.2.5 表达实验标本制作或实验动物操作常用的句型

【常用句型】

- ... was fed/maintained/raised under/with ... 在……条件下饲养
- ... was fasted/starved 6 hours prior to operation 在术前 6 小时禁食
- ... was sacrificed with ... 用……处死
- ... was anesthetized with ... 用……麻醉
- Samples were obtained/taken from ... 标本取自……
- ... was stained with ... 用……染色
- ... was collected/harvested under ... 在……条件下收集
- ... was dehydrated in/by ... 在……条件下脱水

例 16:Venous blood samples of up to 3 mL <u>were collected</u>, and hemoglobin levels <u>were measured</u> with a HemoCue 301＋ device (HemoCue). Serum <u>was separated</u> and <u>frozen</u> for analysis of ferritin and C-reactive protein levels.

采集至少 3 mL 的静脉血样本,用 HemoCue 301＋设备(HemoCue)测量血红蛋白水平。分离并冷冻血清以分析铁蛋白和 C 反应蛋白水平。

例 17:Mice <u>were housed</u> in autoclaved plastic cages with soft woodchip bedding in an air-conditioned room, artificially illuminated daily from 06:00—20:00 hr, and <u>were fed</u> mouse chow and water ad libitum. Mice <u>were injected</u> with propofol, tribromoethanol, urethane, ethanol and pentobarbital in that order at 7- to 10-day intervals.

小鼠被关在铺有柔软木屑的高压灭菌塑料笼子里,配有空调,每天 06:00—20:00 人工照明,并自由饮用食物和水。按 7—10 天间隔给小鼠依次注射异丙酚、三溴乙醇、氨基甲酸乙酯、乙醇和戊巴比妥。

第四节　练习巩固

1. 使用括号里的词汇或短语,将下列材料与方法中出现的句子译成英语。

(1) 病人被诊断出患有心绞痛。(diagnose)

（2）总胆固醇与高密度脂蛋白胆固醇的比率下降不大。（ratio）

（3）我们纳入 921 例严重急性胃肠道出血的患者，并将其中 461 例随机分配接受一种限制性策略。（enroll，assign ... to）

（4）在总数为 66 例次的痉挛中，26 次是用高渗葡萄糖治疗的。（episode）

（5）受伤后第 23 天，尿量平均为 50—100 毫升/24 小时。（average）

（6）对照组年龄平均为 60 岁。（average/mean）

（7）在 150 例接受肾脏移植术的病人中，生存者接受了中位数 1.7 年的随访。（median）

（8）患者每 12 小时分别口服研究药物 150 mg 或 250 mg，共治疗 28 天。（at a dose of）

（9）将 226 例符合研究标准的病人随机分配到一个治疗组。（eligible，assign）

（10）戊巴比妥（Pentobarbital）与生理盐水按照 1∶20 比例稀释，并按 0.24 mL/10 g 进行腹腔内注射。（dilute）

2. 找出下列句子中的错误并加以改正。

（1）At the same time, several ordinary pulmonary function tests were determined.

（2）Eighteen persons had a family history of diabetes mellitus，but only 9 of them were diagnosed as diabetes mellitus by glucose tolerance test.

（3）This article deals with new block therapy of the facial nerve and with the experience in treating 70 cases (including 250 times) of facial spasm.

（4）340 of 5086 patients receiving operations on the extrahepatic biliary trees required reoperations on this system.

（5）It was suggested that among the 12 sufferers，9 of them might receive DMD gene from their mother carriers.

（6）Most of the cases have been performed by means of anastomosis of the superficial temporal artery with the cortical branch of the middle cerebral artery.

（7）The demographic parameters and metabolic profile in 78 hypertensive subjects were compared with 74 normotensives.

（8）Age，waist-to-hip ratio，proinsulin level，hyperglycemia，and dyslipidemia were positively correlated with hypertension. But after adjusted by BMI，this correlation did not exist.

3. 阅读下列论文中的材料与方法节选部分，并分析其语言特征。

Overview and data sources

We studied patterns of commercial air travel out of Guinea，Liberia，and Sierra Leone，the three countries with widespread and intense Ebola virus transmission as of Sept 1，2014，which we deemed the most likely sources of exported infections of Ebola virus. For our travel analyses，we used two complementary datasets from the International Air Transport Association，representing the most up-to-date data currently available. The first dataset includes information on future flight schedules （ie，passenger carrying capacity as seats on flights between directly connected airports），which we used to describe all non-stop flights out of Guinea，Liberia，and Sierra Leone between September 2014，and December 2014. The second dataset includes monthly，passenger-level flight itinerary data from September 2013，to December 2013，which we used to describe the expected final destinations of travellers departing Ebola virus affected countries while accounting for all traveller flight connections.

International air travel out of areas affected by Ebola virus

We first quantified the total volume of international commercial air travellers departing every country in the world in 2013，highlighting Guinea，Liberia，Sierra Leone，the four neighbouring countries that share a land border （Côte d'Ivoire，Guinea-Bissau，Mali，and Senegal），and Nigeria. To estimate how international air traffic flows to and from Guinea，Liberia，and Sierra Leone have changed due to the Ebola epidemic，we calculated the reduction in total aircraft seat capacity based on online media reports of airline flight cancellations and travel restrictions imposed by countries as of Sept 1，2014.

We then analysed the flight itineraries of all international travellers departing Guinea，Liberia，and Sierra Leone between September 2013，and December 2013，and mapped the final destinations of these travellers （ESRI ArcGIS v10），indicating which cities are scheduled to receive non-stop flights between September 2014 and December 2014. We deemed individuals initiating travel from any domestic or international airport within these three countries to have possible exposure to Ebola virus. We deemed all other travellers，including those simply transiting through Guinea，Liberia，or Sierra Leone，or originating from Nigeria or Senegal （where at the time of writing no evidence of widespread community-based transmission was reported), to have no significant risk of exposure to Ebola virus. Although no new cases have been reported in Nigeria since early September, because of the potential for new or undetected cases appearing, we separately assessed global air traffic patterns out of Lagos and Port Harcourt, Nigeria (which collectively include 540 812 travellers, 81% of Nigeria's international air traffic volume in 2013).

We then quantified the number of travellers needed to be screened to capture one traveller potentially exposed to Ebola virus (defined as any individual initiating travel from an airport within Guinea, Liberia, or Sierra Leone) and compared the number of cities in which traveller screening would be required to detect all potentially exposed travellers. This analysis included options for screening at: international points of departure from Guinea, Liberia, or Sierra Leone (exit-screening); international points of arrival on non-stop flights arriving from Guinea, Liberia, or Sierra Leone (entry-screening for direct flights); and international points of arrival via connecting flights (ie, airports receiving travellers via multisegment flights originating from these three countries; entry-screening for indirect flights). To estimate the likelihood of an asymptomatic air traveller infected with Ebola virus (in the incubation period) developing detectable symptomatic illness during the course of an international flight, we calculated the median (IQR) and mean (SD) of travel times for all potential travellers exposed to Ebola virus to reach their final destination. We assumed a 1 h layover for domestic flights and a 2 h layover for international flights.

Projections of international Ebola virus spread

To estimate the potential for international spread of Ebola virus out of Guinea, Liberia, and Sierra Leone via commercial air travel between September 2014 and December 2014, we used the number of active cases (defined as confirmed, probable, or suspected cases within the 21 day period before Sept 21, 2014, as reported by WHO), World Bank 2013 country population estimates, and the monthly number of international outbound air travellers between September 2013 and December 2013 (ie, pre-outbreak flows) to calculate expected numbers of Ebola virus exportations (ie, [number of active cases/country population] × monthly number of international outbound air travellers). We then estimated the expected time in months for one air traveller infected with Ebola virus to depart the above three countries (ie, 1/expected number of Ebola virus exportations per month). This method assumed flows of international travellers before the outbreak (ie, 2013), a homogeneous distribution, and constant prevalence of Ebola virus infection in the general population, an equal risk of infection between travellers and non-travellers, and no under-reporting of cases of Ebola virus. In view of existing uncertainties, we did sensitivity analyses to explore scenarios of increasing case burden ($2\times$, $5\times$, $10\times$), exponential risk in case burden over time, and decreasing international air traffic capacity due to flight cancellations, travel restrictions, or changes in travel behaviours (50%, 75% reduction; appendix).

Traveller destinations and Health System Capacity

As a crude surrogate marker for health-care capacity, we examined the World Bank income group (ie, low-income, lower-middle-income, upper-middle-income, or high income country) of the final destinations of travellers departing Guinea, Liberia, and Sierra Leone. Destination cities of travellers were aggregated to the country level and also compared with selected national indicators of health-care system capacity from the World Bank (eg, health-care expenditures per head, physicians per 1000 people, hospital beds per 1000 people) to identify countries with high levels of connectivity to Ebola virus affected areas but with constrained health-care resources.

第六章 研究结果

第一节 研究结果的功能及主要要求

医学研究一般以定量研究法为主,撰写结果(Results)需要注意以下几个关键方面:

(1) 应以清晰、简洁和客观的方式总结研究的主要发现,而不是罗列全部研究数据,与研究课题无关的数据应予删除;

(2) 应利用文本和图表等呈现数据,对图表的描述必须能清晰地表现研究结果;

(3) 研究的局限性可以在这一部分提及;

(4) 应只是对研究结果的客观陈述,一般无须涉及研究的科学价值和临床意义等内容;

(5) 建议使用子标题组建研究结果,有助于读者理解和定位研究结果;

(6) 结果部分在呈现研究结果时往往不可避免地涉及研究对象、方法、过程等内容,这些内容的技术细节如已经在方法部分得到详尽介绍,结果部分应转换语言表达,避免重复。

结果部分报告数据分析的结果,这些结果与回答特定研究问题紧密有关。其目的是为读者提供在讨论中得出结论所需的所有数据和资料支持。虽然数据的解释应该留给讨论部分,但读者在结果部分结束时仍然应该有足够的信息来确定研究结果是否支持假设,以及它们是否具有学术价值。

结果部分英文表达以过去时书写,是对数据的简明和客观的总结,是对关键研究发现进行有逻辑的呈现。将结果按照与引言和方法部分相同的顺序排列,可以帮助读者理解,并防止读者在阅读论文时感到困惑。对不同的假设或子组分析使用副标题也有助于实现这一点。

此外,不同期刊对论文结果部分的要求会有不同。作者撰写论文意图发表时,应审查并遵循目标期刊的格式指南或指导方针以增加发表的概率。

第二节 研究结果例文分析

下面,我们具体分析一篇著名学术期刊刊登的学术论文的结果部分。

例:

RESULTS

PATIENTS AND FOLLOW-UP

From August 2013 through March 2020, a total of 700 patients were randomly assigned to the PCI group (347 patients) or the optimal-medical-therapy group (353 patients) across 40 centers in the United Kingdom. The trial groups appeared to be well matched in terms of baseline characteristics, medication use, and heart-failure devices, and the trial population was representative of patients with ischemic heart disease and a low ejection fraction in the United Kingdom (Tables 1 and S5 through S7). Among the patients assigned to the PCI group, 334 (96.3%) underwent PCI at a median of 35 days (interquartile range, 15 to 57) after randomization; further planned staged PCI was carried out in 80 patients. The mean British Cardiovascular Intervention Society jeopardy score was 9.3 before the procedure and 2.7 after the procedure (change, -6.6 points; 95% confidence interval [CI], -6.9 to -6.2), which corresponds with an anatomical revascularization index of 71% (95% CI, 67 to 74). Details of the PCI procedures are provided in Table S8. Follow-up concluded in March 2022; the median duration of follow-up was 41 months (interquartile range, 28 to 60) after randomization in both trial groups. Data on the primary outcome were available for 99.1% of the patients (Fig. S1).

PRIMARY OUTCOME AND COMPONENTS

A primary-outcome event of death from any cause or hospitalization for heart failure occurred in 129 patients (37.2%) in the PCI group and in 134 patients (38.0%) in the optimal-medical-therapy group (hazard ratio, 0.99; 95% CI, 0.78 to 1.27, P=0.96) (Table 2 and Fig. 1). A total of 110 patients (31.7%) in the PCI group and 115 patients (32.6%) in the optimal-medical-therapy group died during follow-up (hazard ratio, 0.98; 95% CI, 0.75 to 1.27) (Fig. S2). At least one hospitalization for heart failure occurred in 51 patients (14.7%) in the PCI group and in 54 patients (15.3%) in the optimal-medical-therapy group (hazard ratio, 0.97; 95% CI, 0.66 to 1.43) (Fig. S3). The treatment effect with respect to the primary outcome was consistent across all prespecified subgroups (Figs. 2 and S4 and Table S9).

MAJOR SECONDARY OUTCOMES

The left ventricular ejection fraction changed from baseline by 1.8 percentage points at 6 months and by 2.0 percentage points at 12 months in the PCI group; the corresponding values at 6 and 12 months in the optimal-medical-therapy group were 3.4 and 1.1 percentage points. The left ventricular ejection fraction was similar in the two groups at 6 months (mean difference, −1.6 percentage points; 95% CI, −3.7 to 0.5) and at 12 months (mean difference, 0.9 percentage points; 95% CI, −1.7 to 3.4) (Fig. 3A and Table S10).

The KCCQ overall summary score appeared to favor the PCI group at 6 months (difference in mean scores, 6.5 points; 95% CI, 3.5 to 9.5) and at 12 months (difference in mean scores, 4.5 points; 95% CI, 1.4 to 7.7). The scores in the optimal-medical-therapy group increased over time, and the between-group difference at 24 months was 2.6 points (95% CI, −0.7 to 5.8). Scores across all component domains of the KCCQ appeared to favor the PCI group at 6 months; at 24 months, the mean between-group difference in the quality-of-life domain score was 4.2 points (95% CI, 0.4 to 8.1). Similarly, the scores on the EQ-5D-5L appeared to favor the PCI group at 6 and 12 months, but the difference had diminished at 24 months (Figs. 3B and S5 and Table S11). The distributions of the New York Heart Association functional class and Canadian Cardiovascular Society angina class among the patients were similar in the two groups at baseline and remained similar at 6, 12, and 24 months (Tables S12 and S13).

OTHER SECONDARY OUTCOMES

A total of 250 patients (126 in the PCI group and 124 in the optimal-medical-therapy group) had a heart-failure device implanted before or within 90 days after randomization (Fig. S6). In the PCI group, an ICD was used to terminate ventricular tachycardia or fibrillation at least once in 2 patients (1.8%) at 6 months, in 3 (2.9%) at 12 months, and in 6 (5.9%) at 24 months; the corresponding values in the optimal-medical-therapy group were 4 (3.8%), 7 (6.6%), and 13 (14.0%). The between-group difference in the incidence of appropriate ICD therapy translated to a risk ratio of 0.42 (95% CI, 0.17 to 1.06) at 24 months.

An acute myocardial infarction occurred in 37 patients (10.7%) in the PCI group and in 38 patients (10.8%) in the optimal-medical-therapy group. Although the overall incidence of myocardial infarction was similar in the two groups (hazard ratio, 1.01; 95% CI, 0.64 to 1.60), periprocedural infarction occurred only in the PCI group, and more cases of spontaneous myocardial infarction occurred in the optimal-medicaltherapy group. There were fewer unplanned revascularizations in the PCI group than in the optimal-medical-therapy group (10 [2.9%] vs. 37 [10.5%];

hazard ratio, 0. 27; 95% CI, 0. 13 to 0. 53) (Table S14 and Fig. S7). NT-proBNP levels decreased in both groups at 6 months, but there was no appreciable between-group difference in the levels at any time point (Fig. S8).

A major bleeding episode occurred during the first year in 10 patients (3. 1%) in the PCI group and in 2 patients (0. 6%) in the optimal-medical-therapy group (relative risk, 4. 95; 95% CI, 1. 09 to 22. 43), but there was no substantial difference in the incidence of bleeding at 2 years (relative risk, 1. 42; 95% CI, 0. 55 to 3. 68). A serious adverse event occurred in 102 patients (29. 4%) in the PCI group and in 104 patients (29. 5%) in the optimal medical-therapy group (Table S15).

[Excerpted from Percutaneous revascularization for ischemic left ventricular dysfunction. *N Engl J Med*, 2022, 387(15): 1351 - 1360.]

【分析】

这是《新英格兰医学杂志》2022 年 8 月刊登的一篇学术论文的结果部分。该文探讨了经皮冠状动脉介入治疗(PCI)是否能改善严重缺血性左心室收缩功能障碍患者的无病生存和左心室功能。论文结果是由 4 个部分构成：Patients and Follow-up、Primary Outcome and Components、Major Secondary Outcomes、Other Secondary Outcomes。

第 1 部分 Patients and Follow-up 主要介绍了研究对象病人数、分组情况、病人接受 PCI 操作的相关信息、病人随访以及最终结局数据等。

第 2 部分 Primary Outcome and Components 主要介绍了 PCI 组和最佳药物治疗组患者经历住院或死亡的风险比。

第 3 部分 Major Secondary Outcomes 和第 4 部分 Other Secondary Outcomes 主要介绍了研究中 PCI 组和最佳药物治疗组在其他方面的对比结果，例如：左心室射血分数在时间上的变化、KCCQ 总评分在时间上的变化、ICD 治疗发生率的组间差异、急性心肌梗死发病率、大出血发生率等。

【实用短语】

- randomly assigned to ... group 随机分到……组
- trial groups/population 试验组/试验人群
- ischemic heart disease 缺血性心脏病
- ejection fraction 射血分数
- at a median of 35 days 平均 35 天时
- corresponds with 与……保持一致
- anatomical revascularization index 解剖血管重建指数
- concluded in 在……时间结束
- hospitalization for heart failure 因心脏衰竭住院
- optimal-medical-therapy group 最佳药物治疗组

- difference in mean scores 平均分差异
- ventricular tachycardia or fibrillation 室性心动过速或纤颤
- acute myocardial infarction 急性心肌梗死

【句型模仿】

1. The trial groups appeared to be well matched in terms of baseline characteristics，medication use，and heart-failure devices.

句型"be well matched in terms of"意为"……在……方面是匹配的"，可模仿写作。

2. A primary-outcome event of death from any cause or hospitalization for heart failure occurred in 129 patients（37. 2%）in the PCI group and in 134 patients（38. 0%）in the optimal-medical-therapy group（hazard ratio，0. 99；95% CI，0. 78 to 1. 27，P=0. 96）（Table 2 and Fig. 1）.

句型"... occurred in sb"，表示"某人发生……，某人患上……疾病"等。此句型在本文里多次使用。

3. The left ventricular ejection fraction changed from baseline by 1. 8 percentage points at 6 months and by 2. 0 percentage points at 12 months in the PCI group.

句型"... changed from ... by ＋... % ＋at＋time(时间)in ... "表示变化的幅度或比率，注意介词 "by"的运用。

4. The left ventricular ejection fraction was similar in the two groups at 6 months （mean difference，−1. 6 percentage points；95% CI，−3. 7 to 0. 5）and at 12 months （mean difference，0. 9 percentage points；95% CI，−1. 7 to 3. 4）（Fig. 3A and Table S10）.

The distributions of the New York Heart Association functional class and Canadian Cardiovascular Society angina class among the patients were similar in the two groups at baseline and remained similar at 6，12，and 24 months （Tables S12 and S13）.

句型"... was/were similar in the ... groups ... "表示"……在组别上是相似的/相近的"，此句型在本文里运用频繁。

5. NT-proBNP levels decreased in both groups at 6 months，but there was no appreciable between-group difference in the levels at any time point （Fig. S8）.

... but there was no substantial difference in the incidence of bleeding at 2 years （relative risk，1. 42；95% CI，0. 55 to 3. 68）.

句型"there was no ….. difference in ... "表示"在……方面没有区别或意义"，用于比较。

【长难句理解】

Although the overall incidence of myocardial infarction was similar in the two groups （hazard ratio，1. 01；95% CI，0. 64 to 1. 60），periprocedural infarction occurred only in the PCI group，and more cases of spontaneous myocardial infarction occurred in the optimal-medical therapy group.

这句话较长，是一个主从复合句。Although 引导让步状语从句，主句由 2 个分句构成。让步状语从句中，主语是 "the overall incidence of myocardial infarction（心肌梗死总发生率）"，句型 "be similar in … " 表示"在……方面相似"；主句中的 2 个分句用了同样的句型 "… occur in … "，表示"发生了……"。译文：尽管两组的心肌梗死总发生率相似（风险比，1.01；95% CI, 0.64—1.60），但 PCI 组发生了围手术期梗死，而最佳药物治疗组发生了较多的自发性心肌梗死病例。

第三节　研究结果的语言特征与常用句型

3.1　结果部分时态的选择

结果部分叙述的是在论文撰写之前就已经完成的实验结果，用于描述当前研究中已获得的结果，建议使用一般过去时态叙述得到的结果。

例 1：

Patients

Of 126 patients screened，95 were enrolled：47 were assigned to the IVIG group and 48 to the placebo group (Fig. 1). A total of 45 patients（96%）in the IVIG group and 46 patients（96%）in the placebo group completed the randomized, placebo-controlled phase of the trial and continued to the open-label extension phase (reasons for exclusions are given in Fig. 1). A total of 34 patients（72%）in the IVIG group and 35 patients（73%）in the placebo group completed the extension phase up to week 40. During the placebo controlled phase，5 patients in the placebo group crossed over to receive IVIG（2 patients were switched because of confirmed deterioration and 3 patients were switched in error）；no patient in the IVIG group crossed over to receive placebo. Data on the primary and secondary end points were missing for 2 patients in each trial group. In total，664 infusion cycles of IVIG were administered at a median dose of 2.0 g per kilogram over a median of 2.4 infusion days per cycle. The safety analysis during the placebo controlled phase included 52 patients who received IVIG and 48 patients who received placebo，and the safety analysis during the open-label extension phase included 95 patients who received IVIG.

[Excerpted from Trial of Intravenous Immune Globulin in Dermatomyositis. *N Engl J Med*, 2023，388(1)：94.]

【分析】

这一段落节选自一篇论文的结果部分,介绍参与研究的样本情况。很明显,句中动词 were enrolled、were assigned、completed、continued、were switched、crossed over、were missing、were administered、included、received 等全部使用一般过去时。

例 2:

Colonoscopy Screening

The percentage of participants who <u>underwent</u> screening varied among the countries (from 33.0% in Poland to 60.7% in Norway) and <u>was higher</u> overall among men than among women and among older participants than among younger participants (Table 1). The cecum <u>was intubated</u> in 96.8% of the colonoscopies performed, and the quality of bowel preparation <u>was adequate</u> in more than 90% of the colonoscopies. Colorectal cancer <u>was diagnosed</u> at screening in 62 participants (0.5% of those who underwent screening). These 62 cases <u>included</u> 2 cases in Poland that had been classified as adenomas in our previous analysis (see the Supplementary Appendix). Adenomas <u>were detected and removed</u> at screening in 3634 participants (30.7% of those who underwent screening). A total of 15 participants (0.13%) <u>had</u> polypectomy-related major bleeding; all cases of bleeding <u>were treated</u> endoscopically and <u>did not warrant</u> further interventions (Table 1). No perforations or screening-related deaths <u>occurred</u> within 30 days after screening.

[Excerpted from Effect of Colonoscopy Screening on Risks of Colorectal Cancer and Related Death. *N Engl J Med*, 2022, 387(17): 1547 - 1556.]

【分析】

这一段落节选自《新英格兰医学杂志》,介绍了肠镜筛查结直肠癌症的结果。显然,句中动词 underwent、was higher、was intubated、was adequate、was diagnosed、included、were detected and removed、had、were treated、did not warrant、occurred 等都使用了一般过去时。

不是阐述实验结果,而是说明表注、图注的内容、数据、符号时,用一般现在时表达。

例 3：

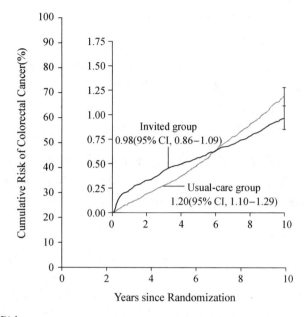

Figure 1　Cumulative Risk of Colorectal Cancer at 10 Years in Intertion-to-Screen Analyses
The inset shows the same data on an enlarged y axis. I bars indicate 95％ confidence intervals.

［Excerpted from Effect of Colonoscopy Screening on Risks of Colorectal Cancer and Related Death. *N Engl J Med*，2022，387(17)：1547 - 1556.］

【分析】

上面 Figure 1 下方的图注说明"The inset shows the same data on an enlarged y axis. I bars indicate 95％ confidence intervals"中动词 show 和 indicate 都使用了一般现在时。

例 4：

（1）Details of the PCI procedures are provided in Table S8.

（2）A total of 45 patients（96％）in the IVIG group and 46 patients（96％）in the placebo group completed the phase of the trial and continued to the open-label extension phase（reasons for exclusions are given in Fig. 1）.

【分析】

用文字来描述图表展示的研究数据时,可用此类句型"… is/are provided/shown/given in Table … /Figure … "来表达,一般动词用一般现在时,如上面句子中的"are provided,are given"。

例 5：<u>Table 2 shows</u> the incidence of adverse events per admission according to demographic characteristics and insurance type.

【分析】

使用句型"Table … /Figure … show/provide/indicate … "描述文中图表时,常用一般现在时表达,如本句中"Table 2 shows"就是此类用法。

3.2 结果部分常用的句型

结果部分的研究结果除了用文本来描述外,尽量用图表来表现,通过图表本身逻辑让读者了解研究的发现。以研究数据为基础,以可视化为手段,目的是清晰描述论文的实验结果,支持论文提出的观点。一般常用的核心句式分类如下:

3.2.1 描写研究目的或步骤

【常用句型】

• Changes in X and Y were compared using … 使用……比较 X 和 Y 的变化

• The first set of analyses examined the impact of … 第一组分析考察了……的影响

• The correlation between X and Y was tested using … 运用……检测 X 和 Y 之间的相关性

• The average scores of X and Y were compared in order to … 比较 X 和 Y 的平均得分以便……

例 6：<u>A</u> semi-parametric joint frailty <u>model was used for</u> the analysis of the outcome of the first and subsequent hospitalizations for any cause.

采用半参数关节衰弱模型分析任何原因导致的首次和后续住院的情况。

例 7：All six sensitivity <u>analyses showed treatment differences</u> consistent with the primary analysis, and there were no indications of effect by sex or age group (Fig. S2 and Table S2 in the Supplementary Appendix).

所有六项敏感性分析显示治疗差异与初步分析一致,并且没有性别或年龄组影响的迹象(补充附录中的图 S2 和表 S2)。

3.2.2 描写表格或图表

【常用句型】

• Figure 1 shows/presents/provides/compares … an overview of … /the experimental data on … /the intercorrelations among … /the results obtained from … /preliminary analysis of …

图 1 显示(展示/提供/比较)……的概述/关于……的实验数据/……之间的相互关系/从……得到的结果/……的初步分析

• The table below/The pie chart above … illustrates/shows/provides/…

下面的表格/上面的饼状图/说明/显示……

• As shown in Figure 1/As can be seen from the table above/From the graph above … , the X group reported … .

如图 1 所示/从上面的表格中可以看出/从上面的图表中，X 组报告……

• The results of … /The results obtained from … be shown/be seen/be presented/be compared/be given … in Table 1/Figure 1

表 1/图 1 可以显示/展示/比较……的结果/从……得到的结果

例 8：Table S10 provides details of the observed between-group differences in hematocrit and hemoglobin levels and the absence of clinically relevant differences in blood calcium，phosphate，and sodium levels，as assessed in a subgroup of patients at 18 months.

表 S10 详细说明了 18 个月时在亚组患者中观察到的血细胞比容和血红蛋白水平的组间差异，而血钙、血磷和血钠水平无相关临床差异。

例 9：Examples of adverse events，including severity category and preventability assessment，are given in Table S8.

表 S8 列举了一些不良事件的例子（包括严重程度分类和可预防性评估）。

3.2.3　描写肯定或否定结果

【常用句型】

• The mean score for X was … X 的平均分数是……

• A two-way ANOVA revealed that … 双向方差分析显示……

• This result is significant at the p＝0.05 level. 该结果在 p＝0.05 水平上具有显著性。

• A positive correlation was found between X and Y. X 与 Y 呈正相关。

• There was a significant difference in X （p＜0.01）… X 有显著性差异（p＜0.01）。

• No significant difference/correlation was found between … /compared with … 与……相比/……之间没有显著差异/相关性。

例 10：At 24 months，the mean between-group difference in the quality-of-life domain score was 4.2 points （95％ CI，0.4 to 8.1）.

24 个月时，生活质量领域评分的平均组间差异为 4.2 分（95％ CI，0.4—8.1）。

例 11：A major bleeding episode occurred during the first year in 10 patients （3.1％）in the PCI group and in 2 patients （0.6％）in the optimal-medical-therapy group （relative risk，4.95；95％ CI，1.09 to 22.43），but there was no substantial difference in the incidence of bleeding at 2 years （relative risk，1.42；95％ CI，0.55 to

3.68).

    PCI 组 10 例患者(3.1%)和最佳药物治疗组 2 例患者(0.6%)在第 1 年内发生了大出血事件(相对危险度,4.95;95% CI, 1.09—22.43),但 2 年内的出血发生率无显著差异(相对危险度,1.42; 95% CI, 0.55—3.68)。

3.2.4　描写调查或访谈涉及的比例

【常用句型】

- Over half of those surveyed reported that ...　超过一半的被调查者报告说……
- A minority/majority of participants (17%/92%) indicated that ...
少数/大多数参与者(17%/92%)表示……
- 70% of those who were interviewed indicated that ...　70%的受访者表示……
- Almost two-thirds of the participants (64%) said/commented that ...　几乎三分之二的参与者(64%)表示/评论……

    例 12:Among all admissions, 523 (18.6%) involved at least one adverse event that was categorized as significant (i. e., caused unnecessary harm but resulted in rapid recovery), 211 (7.5%) involved a serious adverse event (as defined above), 34 (1.2%) included at least one adverse event that was life-threatening, and 7 (0.2%) involved an adverse event that was fatal.

    在所有住院患者中,523 例(18.6%)涉及至少 1 起显著的不良事件(即造成不必要的伤害,但患者快速康复),211 例(7.5%)涉及严重不良事件(如上文定义),34 例(1.2%)包括至少 1 起危及生命的不良事件,7 例(0.2%)涉及致死性不良事件。

3.3　结果部分单词选择技巧

    使用简洁而客观的动词来描述结果,如 show、indicate、demonstrate、highlight、identify、detect、observe、find、report、confirm 等。

    减少否定句,特别是主要起修辞作用的双重否定句,使意思更加明白流畅。否定词可用含有否定意义的词汇或词组代替,例如:little、few、no、without、fail 等。

    尤其值得注意的是,减少使用主观色彩浓厚的态度副词以强调结果的重要性,例如 really、obviously、clearly、significantly、certainly、incredibly 等。

第四节 研究结果中的常用图表

4.1 论文中图表的重要性

图表是研究论文的重要组成部分,它们提供了支持研究结论的研究结果、统计数据和相关信息,结构完整、简洁自明。

图表在结果部分的重要性:

• 可视化表示(visual representation):图表将不易理解和解释的数据可视化,帮助读者快速掌握研究结果的要点,并得出自己的结论。

• 组织数据(organizing data):图表有助于以系统化和结构化的方式组织大量数据,使读者更容易识别数据中的模式和趋势。

• 清晰和准确(clarity and accuracy):图表允许研究人员以清晰和准确的方式呈现数据。它们可以包括精确的数字、百分比和其他难以用文字形式表达的信息。

• 比较(comparison):图表允许在不同的数据集或组之间进行比较,可使读者更容易识别异同,并从数据中得出有意义的结论。

• 效率(efficiency):图表可以更有效地利用研究论文中的空间,可以以紧凑简洁的格式传达大量的信息,节省空间,使研究论文更具可读性。

4.2 常见图表类型

4.2.1 描述性表格

描述性表格(descriptive tables)提供研究中收集的数据的摘要。它们通常用于表示基本的描述性统计,如平均值、中位数、标准差和频率。例如:

Descriptive Statistics

	N Statistic	Mean Statistic	Std. Deviation Statistic	Skewness	
				Statistic	Std. Error
Reaction time (milliseconds)-no alcohol-trial 1	36	753.00	60.836	−.868	.393
Reaction time (milliseconds)-no alcohol-trial 2	36	767.42	67.530	−1.046	.393
Reaction time (milliseconds)-no alcohol-trial 3	36	782.72	77.249	−.401	.393

	N Statistic	Mean Statistic	Std. Deviation Statistic	Skewness	
				Statistic	Std. Error
Reaction time （milliseconds）-no alcohol-trial 4	36	797.67	79.690	−.418	.393
Reaction time （milliseconds）-no alcohol-trial 5	36	813.97	82.198	−.624	.393
Valid N (listwise)	36				

4.2.2 比较表格

比较表格（comparative tables）用于显示两个或多个组之间的差异,或用于比较不同变量的结果。例如：

Knowledge	Mean±SD		
	Group A （n=102）	Group B （n=98）	Group C （n=107）
Dose of drug	0.34±0.47	0.37±0.5	0.43±0.5
Mechanism of action	0.23±0.4	0.26±0.4	0.31±0.5
Adverse effect	0.47±0.5	0.53±0.5	0.64±0.4
Precautions for use	0.11±0.3	0.17±0.4	0.23±0.4
Contraindication for use	0.20±0.4	0.25±0.4	0.28±0.4
Aware about complication	0.74±0.4	0.73±0.4	0.82±0.3
Total score	2.10±1.1	2.32±1.2	2.72±1.2*,**

ANOVA test. * $P < 0.05$ as compared to Group B in Group C, ** $P < 0.001$ as compared to Group A in Group C.

ANOVA：Analysis of variance,SD：Standard deviation

4.2.3 相关表格

相关表格（correlation tables）显示变量之间的相关系数,也可以显示回归分析的结果。例如：

Correlations

Pearson Correlation

	Wechsel IQ Test Score	Depression Test Score	Anxiety Test Score Social
Wechsel IQ Test Score	1	082	378 **
Depression Test Score	082	1	222 *
Anxiety Test Score	378 **	222 *	1
Social Functioning Test Score	−.077	−.328 **	−.405 **
General Well Being Test Score	−.037	−.801 **	−.226 *

** Correlation is significant at the 0.01 level (2-tailed)

* Correlation is significant at the 0.05 level (2-tailed)

4.2.4 纵向表格

纵向表格(longitudinal tables)用于显示变量的变化。它们可能显示重复测量分析或纵向回归分析的结果。

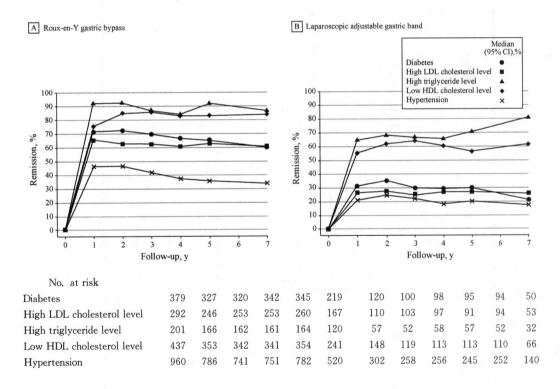

4.2.5 定性表格

定性表格(qualitative tables)用于总结定性数据,如访谈记录或开放式调查反馈。它们可能呈现从数据中产生的主题或类别。例如:

Research method	Participants	Data collection	Data capturing	Data treatment	Data analysis
A. Ethnography	Wards	• Care participant observation • 3 wards • 45 hours	• Field journal	• Interpreting field notes • Triangulating with B and C	Observational data were examined and interpreted for common themes
B. Narrative	Nurses	• Free Association Narrative Interviews • 16 nurse participants • 14.9 hours	• Digital voice recorder • Research journal	• Transcription • Triangulating with A and C	Narrative data were examined and interpreted for common themes until saturation reached
C. Narrative	Residents	• Intersubjectivity informed therapeutic interactions • 10 resident participants • 59 hours	• Digital voice recorder • Research journal	• Transcription • Triangulating with A and B	Narrative data were examined and interpreted for common themes until saturation reached

4.2.6 统计图

统计图(statistical charts)统计图是利用点、线、面、体等绘制成几何图形,以表示各种数量间的关系及其变动情况的工具。常见的统计图主要有:柱状图(bar chart)、饼图(pie chart)、XY 散点图(X,Y scatterplot)、线图(line graph)、流式图(flow cytometry)等,科学期刊对此类统计图要求严格,每种类型的统计图都有许多细节需要注意。具体图例,请参考下面几种统计图。

- 柱状图

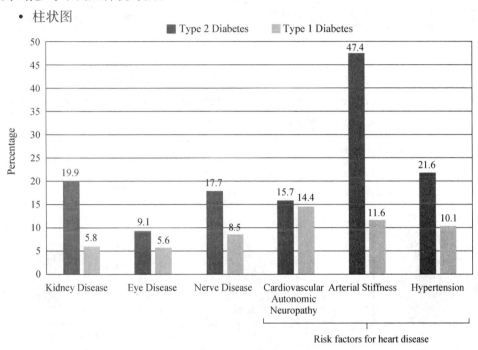

Figure 1 Percentage of young adults with diabetes developing complications from the disease

- 散点图

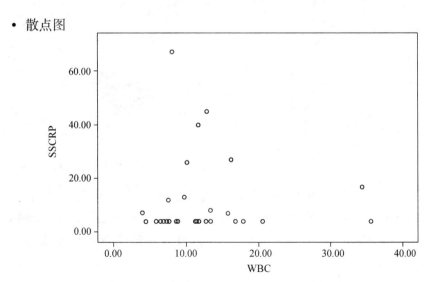

Figure 1 Scatter plot for correlation between C-reactive protein and white blood cell in asymptomatic steady state hemoglobin SS group($P=0.73$)

- 线图

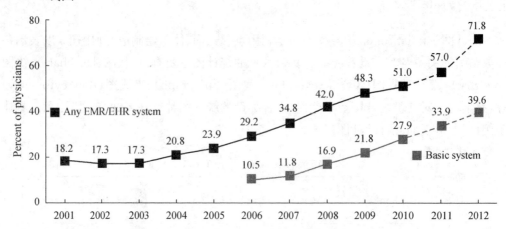

Figure 2　Percentage of office-based physicians with EMR/EHR systems：United States，2001—2010 and preliminary 2011—2012

- 流式细胞术散点图

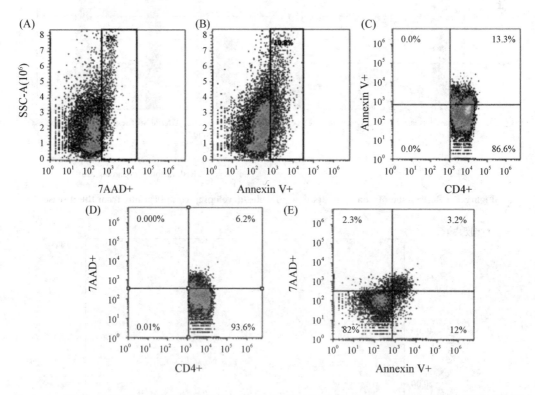

　　• 照片（photos）：医学照片经常出现在医学论文中。常见的照片主要指 X-ray、CT、PET-CT、MRI 等造影照片。照片应遵照真实性原则，可以适当调整整体亮度、对比度等，但不能进行 PS 调整。同时，可以用箭头指示病变部位。例如 MRI 照片：

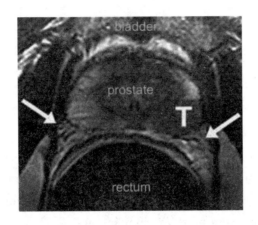

- 组织切片染色图

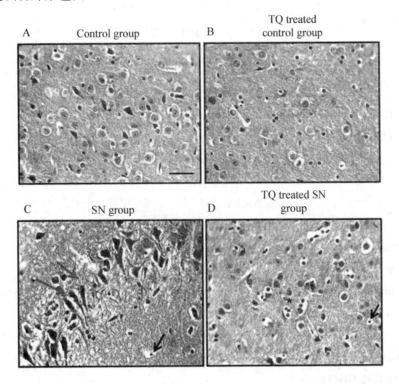

　　结果部分撰写完后,自己审核,回顾论文的前言和方法,确保无遗漏或冗余。同时,可邀请项目组其他成员审阅讨论,以便进一步完善,同时,也为撰写讨论部分做好准备。

第五节 练习巩固

阅读下列医学论文的结果部分，完成以下练习。

RESULTS

DEMOGRAPHICS

Among US women aged 15 - 49 who had a first singleton birth in 2017（n＝1,428,184），0.3％（n＝4,412）had HCV（Table 1）. Furthermore, 8.2％（n＝116,764）of singleton births were preterm. Few infants（7.7％, n＝109,064）had either low or very low birth weight, and few full-term infants had a low or intermediate Apgar score（2.5％; n＝34,832）. White women had a higher prevalence of HCV infection（0.4％; n＝3,909）compared to Black women（0.1％; n＝222）（Table 2）. Infants born to Black women, as compared to infants born to White women, had higher prevalence of preterm birth（11.1％ v 7.7％）, very low（2.9％ v 1.1％）and low（9.9％ v 5.4％）infant birth weight, and low（1.3％ v 0.6％）and intermediate（2.4％ v 1.7％）Apgar scores.

BIRTH WEIGHT

On average, infants born to women who had HCV were 175.5 g lighter in unadjusted linear regression modeling（95％ CI: −192.53, −158.43）and were 42.0 g lighter in the adjusted linear regression modeling（95％ CI: −58.81, −25.30）, as compared to women who did not have HCV, among all births（Table 3）. Among White women, infants were 64.6 g lighter in adjusted models（95％ CI: −81.91, −47.26）if their mother had an HCV infection. Among Black women, in the adjusted model, infants were 80.3 g lighter if their mother had an HCV infection but this was not statistically significant（95％ CI: −162.48, 1.93）. HCV infection may have a greater impact on birth weight of infants born to Black women as compared to White women but this difference did not rise to statistical significance.

PRETERM BIRTH

For all singleton births, maternal HCV infection increased the odds of having a preterm birth in both the unadjusted（OR: 1.69; 95％ CI: 1.54, 1.85）and adjusted logistic regression models（OR: 1.06; 95％ CI: 0.96, 1.17）（Table 4）. With adjustment, the odds of having a preterm birth among HCV infected women was reduced compared to the unadjusted model and was no longer statistically significant.

Among HCV-infected White women, the odds of having a preterm birth was similar to the non-stratified model for both the unadjusted（OR: 1.78; 95％ CI: 1.61, 1.96）and adjusted models（OR: 1.06; 95％ CI: 0.96, 1.18）. Black women who had an HCV infection had a higher odds of preterm birth when compared to their uninfected counterparts in both the unadjusted (OR: 1.74; 95% CI: 1.22, 2.50) and adjusted models (OR: 1.35; 95% CI: 0.93, 1.97). Comparing the effect estimates for adjusted models, HCV-infected Black women have a higher odds of preterm birth than HCV-infected White women when compared to their uninfected counterparts. However, this difference was not statistically significant.

APGAR SCORE

When examining all singleton full term births, maternal HCV infection was significantly associated with low or intermediate Apgar score in the unadjusted (OR: 1.55; 95% CI: 1.27, 1.90) and adjusted logistic regression models (OR: 1.26; 95% CI: 1.03, 1.55) (Table 5). Upon stratification, for White women this same association was observed in the unadjusted model (OR: 1.52; 95% CI: 1.22, 1.89) and the adjusted model (OR: 1.23; 95% CI: 0.98, 1.53). Among Black women, the association between maternal HCV infection and low and intermediate Apgar score had a similar magnitude and direction in the unadjusted (OR: 1.33; 95% CI: 0.55, 3.25) and adjusted models (OR: 1.24; 95% CI: 0.51, 3.02). The association between maternal HCV infection and low and intermediate Apgar score was similar across the race stratified adjusted models。

SENSITIVITY ANALYSIS -LMP ESTIMATES

When using the LMP method rather than the OE method to estimate gestational age, the association between maternal HCV infection and preterm birth from both logistic regression models are similar to estimates obtained using the OE method (Supplemental Table 1). Additionally, for White women, the associations were similar to the results using the OE method. Among Black women, the association between maternal HCV infection and preterm birth decreased in both models. However, the adjusted estimate was still higher among Black women than White women.

1. 请把上面例文中的实用短语翻译成合适的中文。

(1) a first singleton birth

(2) full term infants

(3) a higher prevalence of HCV infection

(4) preterm birth

(5) birth weight of infants

(6) Apgar Score

(7) demographics

(8) sensitivity analysis

2. 请根据本章内容的学习，分析上面 Results 内容的结构特征和语言特征。

3. 根据上面学术论文的 Results 内容，撰写该论文摘要（Abstract）中的 Results 部分，字数控制在 200 字以内。

第七章 讨 论

第一节 讨论的主要内容

讨论部分(Discussion)是医学论文中最为关键,也是提炼和升华研究价值和意义的一节。这部分不仅要对自己的研究结果进行深入分析,还要旁征博引,与引用的文献报道的结果或讨论对比结合起来,这样才能论述严密,同时令人信服。此外,讨论部分也需对本研究工作的缺陷或不足做出解释与评价,并说明有待解决的问题和以后研究的方向。因此,讨论部分可以说是整篇论文中较为难写的一个部分,也往往是编辑或评阅人判定论文能否发表的一个重要标准。

不同国际期刊在"作者须知"(Instructions for Authors)中都明确了讨论部分的写作要求。例如期刊 *Virology* 对讨论部分的写作要求为:"The Discussion should provide an interpretation of the results in relation to previously published work and to the experimental system at hand and should not contain extensive repetition of the Results section or reiteration of the Introduction. In short papers, the Results and Discussion sections may be combined."期刊 *PLOS Medicine* 对讨论部分的写作要求为:"The discussion should be concise and tightly argued. It should start with a brief summary of the main findings. It should include paragraphs on the generalisability, clinical relevance, strengths, and, most importantly, the limitations of your study. You may wish to discuss the following points also. How do the conclusions affect the existing knowledge in the field? How can future research build on these observations? What are the key experiments that must be done?"从这些要求可以看出,大部分期刊都希望投稿人在写作讨论时至少要做到以下几点:

(1)讨论部分不能简单重复结果或前言部分的内容,而必须对研究的主要结果做一总结;

(2)研究的局限性和未来研究方向需要在讨论部分有所涉及;

(3)写作语言应做到深入浅出、简洁扼要,避免无根据地扩大研究讨论的范围,也要避免和讨论与实验结果无关或不一致的内容。

第二节 讨论例文分析

下面,我们具体分析学术论文的讨论部分写作。

例:

Discussion

We evaluated the effect of adding eplerenone to recommended treatment for systolic heart failure in patients with mild symptoms (NYHA functional class II symptoms). The rate of the primary outcome, a composite of death from cardiovascular causes or hospitalization for heart failure, was 18.3% in the eplerenone group versus 25.9% in the placebo group. This effect of eplerenone was consistent across all prespecified subgroups. With eplerenone, there was also a reduction in both the rate of death from any cause and the rate of hospitalization for any reason.

The mechanisms by which mineralocorticoid-receptor antagonists such as eplerenone provide cardiovascular protection in patients with heart failure are not completely understood. Activation of the mineralocorticoid receptor by both aldosterone and cortisol plays an important role in the pathophysiology of heart failure, and mineralocorticoid receptors are overexpressed in the failing heart. Despite therapy with ACE inhibitors, ARBs, and beta-blockers, patients with even mildheart failure may have persistently elevated plasma aldosterone and cortisol levels. Mineralocorticoid receptors are not blocked by these treatments.

Activation of the mineralocorticoid receptor has been shown to promote cardiac fibrosis in experimental models. In patients with heart failure, as well as in patients after myocardial infarction, the use of mineralocorticoid-receptor antagonists decreases extracellular-matrix turnover, as assessed by measuring serum levels of collagen biomarkers. Experimental and clinical studies suggest that mineralocorticoid-receptor antagonists favorably affect several other important mechanisms known to have a role in the progression of heart failure.

In our study, as anticipated, there was an increased incidence of hyperkalemia among patients receiving eplerenone. This finding underscores the need to measure serum potassium levels serially and to adjust the dose of eplerenone accordingly. We attempted to minimize the risk of hyperkalemia by excluding patients with a baseline serum potassium level above 5.0 mmol per liter and a baseline estimated GFR below 30 ml per minute per 1.73 m^2.

In contrast, the risk of hypokalemia was significantly reduced among patients receiving eplerenone. This is important because a serum potassium level below 4.0 mmol per liter has been associated with an increased risk of death from any cause among patients with systolic heart failure.

Our study has some limitations. Our results may not be applicable to all patients with mild symptoms, because to be eligible for the study, patients had to have additional factors known to increase cardiovascular risk, including an age over 55 years, in most cases an ejection fraction of no more than 30%, and a recent hospitalization for a cardiovascular reason. Use of an implantable cardioverter-defibrillator was relatively infrequent, but this finding is similar to those in recent registries and trials. The early stopping of the trial may have resulted in overestimation of the magnitude of the treatment effect, but the results are consistent with those seen in RALES.

In conclusion, our study showed that, as compared with placebo, eplerenone added to recommended therapy for systolic heart failure in patients with mild symptoms was associated with a reduction in the rate of death from a cardiovascular cause or hospitalization for heart failure. Similar reductions were seen in rates of death from any cause, death from cardiovascular causes, hospitalization for any reason, and hospitalization for heart failure.

[Excerpted from Eplerenone in Patients with Systolic Heart Failure and Mild Symptoms. *N Engl J Med*, 2011, 364(1):11-21.]

【分析】

这是一篇关于收缩期心衰和有轻微症状的病人使用强心剂（Eplerenone，中文名依普利酮）的讨论论文。作者共分为7个自然段进行讨论，前5个自然段分析讨论依普利酮和安慰剂相比，能够降低有轻微症状（NYHA功能Ⅱ类症状）的收缩期心力衰竭患者的住院率和死亡率，其中第2、3段对治疗原理进行讨论，第4、5段对治疗引起的副作用——高钾血症进行讨论。而在第6段，作者开始讨论本研究的局限，这是讨论部分中重要的一个内容。最后一个自然段，是论文的结论部分，作者运用简洁的语言，将全文研究进行了总结，即再次重申依普利酮对于轻微症状的收缩期心力衰竭患者的效用。

【实用短语】

- recommended treatment for 推荐疗法
- with mild symptoms 症状轻微
- promote cardiac fibrosis 加重心脏纤维化
- an increased incidence of hyperkalemia 高钾血症发病率增加
- measure serum potassium levels serially 连续测量血清钾水平
- adjust the dose accordingly 相应调整剂量
- minimize the risk of 将风险最小化

- be eligible for 符合入选条件

【句型模仿】

1. We <u>evaluated the effect</u> of adding eplerenone to <u>recommended treatment</u> for systolic heart failure in <u>patients with</u> mild symptoms (NYHA functional class Ⅱ symptoms).

请注意本句中"评估疗效"（evaluated the effect）、"在推荐疗法中加入……药物"（add ... to recommended treatment）以及"患有某种疾病的患者（patients with ＋疾病名称）"的表达方法。

2. The <u>mechanisms by which</u> mineralocorticoid-receptor antagonists such as eplerenone provide cardiovascular protection in patients with heart failure <u>are not completely understood.</u>

本句中"The mechanisms by which ... are not completely understood"意为"发挥疗效的机制尚未被充分理解"，主语为 mechanisms，而后借助定语从句进行描述，结构紧凑。

3. In our study, as anticipated, there was <u>an increased incidence of</u> hyperkalemia among patients receiving eplerenone. This finding <u>underscores the need</u> to measure serum potassium levels serially and to adjust the dose of eplerenone accordingly.

本句中"an increased incidence of"意为"升高的发病率"，"underscores the need to ..."意为"强调……的需要"。

【长难句理解】

1. Activation of the mineralocorticoid receptor by both aldosterone and cortisol plays an important role in the pathophysiology of heart failure, and mineralocorticoid receptors are overexpressed in the failing heart.

醛固酮和皮质醇对盐皮质激素受体的激活在心力衰竭的病理生理中起着重要作用，心脏衰竭时，盐皮质激素受体过度表达。

2. Our results may not be applicable to all patients with mild symptoms, because to be eligible for the study, patients had to have additional factors known to increase cardiovascular risk, including an age over 55 years, in most cases an ejection fraction of no more than 30％, and a recent hospitalization for a cardiovascular reason.

我们的结果可能并不适用于所有轻微症状的患者，因为要符合研究条件，患者必须有其他已知的增加心血管风险的因素，包括年龄超过 55 岁，在大多数情况下射血分数不超过 30％，以及最近因心血管原因住院。

第三节　讨论的语言特征与常用句型

"讨论"作为医学学术论文的一项重要组成部分,在英文表达上有其特殊的时态运用和一些常见的表达句型。下面逐一进行分析。

3.1　讨论部分时态的运用

讨论部分中使用的时态依具体内容而异。首先,涉及背景说明的部分一般用一般现在时或现在完成时,描述、介绍别人在相关领域的研究成果时可用一般过去时。

例 1：More than a decade <u>has passed</u> since the last *Lancet* Seminar on depression in adolescents, and during this time its prevalence <u>has sharply increased</u>, especially in females during late adolescence and early adult life.

自上次《柳叶刀》青少年抑郁症研讨会以来,已经过去了十多年,在此期间,抑郁症患病率急剧上升,特别是在青春期晚期和成年早期的女性中。

例 2：To date, <u>there have been</u> 14 genetic mutations linked to MODY. The most common forms of MODY are HNF1A MODY-3 and GCK MODY-2 gene mutations and result in abnormal vesicle packaging or release of insulin, which leads to a milder form of diabetes.

迄今为止,已有 14 种基因突变与青年发病的成年型糖尿病(MODY)有关。最常见的 MODY 形式是 HNF1A MODY-3 和 GCK MODY-2 基因突变,导致囊泡异常包装或胰岛素释放,从而导致轻度糖尿病。

其次,在描述将结果推广成一般理论这一过程时,要注意时态的运用。如果研究者认为研究结论只适于本研究环境和条件时,就使用一般过去时进行表达,而研究者认为该研究结论具有普遍意义时,可用一般现在时或一般将来时。一般来说,使用一般现在时态进行叙述的情况要多一些。

例 3：Appropriate treatment and proper management of the atypical forms of diabetes are contingent upon the correct diagnoses. <u>The authors recommend</u> keeping an open mind when diagnosing diabetes to avoid misdiagnosis. Additional investigation should be considered if standard treatment is ineffective.

适当治疗和正确管理非典型糖尿病取决于正确的诊断。作者建议在诊断糖尿病时保持开放的心态,以避免误诊。如果标准治疗无效,应考虑进一步调查。

例 4：<u>In conclusion, depression is highly heterogeneous</u>, more so in young people, and spans a spectrum of severity. Neuroscience and genetic discoveries coupled with social and clinical data could be used to personalise treatment and improve outcomes.

总之,抑郁症是高度异质性的,在年轻人中更是如此,并且严重程度不一。结合社会和临床数据,神经科学和遗传学发现可以用于个性化治疗和改善结局。

3.2 讨论部分的常用句型

3.2.1 对已汇报的实验结果进行再次总结陈述的句型

【常用句型】

- There was no significant difference in … between … group and … group.
- … was higher/lower in … group than in … group.
- We found that … /It was found that …
- … was/were found to do/to have done …
- … , as has been suggested/indicated.
- We hypothesized that …

例 5:In the present study, we observed large phenotypic variation within the outbred mice even when a small number of mice (10 mice of each sex) was examined.

在本研究中,我们观察到即使在对少量小鼠(雌雄各 10 只)进行检查时,杂交小鼠内部也存在较大的表型变异。

例 6:There has been much progress, but countless questions circling the concept of depression and its origins still remain unanswered.

研究已经取得了很大的进展,但围绕抑郁症的概念及其起源的无数问题仍然没有答案。

3.2.2 将研究成果推广成一般理论的主要句型

【常用句型】

- In conclusion/summary,…
- Our findings provide support for …
- Our findings suggest/indicate that …

例 7:Our present study clearly shows that phenotypic variation within commercial outbred ICR mice is not small as had been speculated, but rather is large, at least for the drugs that depress central nervous system.

我们目前的研究清楚地表明,商业性的杂交 ICR(Institute of Cancer Research)小鼠的表型变异并不像之前推测的那样小,而是很大,至少对于抑制中枢神经系统的药物来说是这样的。

例 8:These findings support a call for action for quality and safety committees to improve hygiene curriculum and provider attire guidelines.

这些发现支持了质量和安全委员会采取行动,以改进卫生学课程、指导医护人员着装。

3.2.3 介绍本研究的优势及益处的主要句型

【常用句型】
- This study has some strengths/advantages/benefits. First,... Second,...
- These findings can be applied to ...
- These findings can be used to ...
- These findings benefit ... /are beneficial for ...

例 9:This review has several implications for clinical practice and public policy.
这篇综述对临床实践和公共政策有几点影响。

例 10:The suggestions outlined in this article, based on available evidence, may serve as a guideline for health care professionals and hospital systems to reduce the spread of bacterial pathogens, including MDROs, that have the potential to precipitate hospital-acquired infections.
本文根据现有证据概述的建议可作为卫生保健专业人员和医院系统减少细菌病原体(包括耐多药抗药性药物)传播的指南,这些病原体有可能引发医院获得性感染。

3.2.4 介绍本研究的局限性的主要句型

【常用句型】
- This study has some limitations. First,... Second,...
- ... is/are limited by ...
- Despite ... , there still has ...

例 11:This systematic review is not without limitations. Each study provides its own set of guidance based on author opinion/rationale, practical considerations, and evidence of relatively low power. Differences also existed in methodology for culturing and sampling attire with studies searching for and targeting a variable set of isolates. There remains need for more robust research regarding potentially pathogenic bacterial transmission through HCW attire.
这篇系统性综述并非没有局限性。基于作者的观点/理论基础、实际考虑和相对低效力的证据,每项研究都提供了自己的一套指导。在培养和取样的方法上也存在差异,因为研究寻找和针对的是一组可变的分离株。对于发现通过医护人员(healthcare worker,HCW)服装传播的潜在致病性细菌,仍需要进行更有力的研究。

例 12:Despite this progress, research has yet to address several issues, almost consistently identified as important.

尽管取得了这些进展,但研究尚未解决几个问题,这几个问题几乎一直被认为是重要的。

3.2.5 介绍本领域未来研究方向的主要句型

【常用句型】

- In future studies, we should ...
- Further studies should focus on ...
- This area of ... requires/needs further studies.

例 13: There are many issues to be addressed in future research, and the preceding sections pointed to several directions. Rather than reiterate these here, this section will briefly outline three issues that it is hoped future research will address.

在未来的研究中有许多问题需要解决,前面的章节指出了几个方向。在此不再重申,本节将简要概述三个问题,希望未来的研究将解决这些问题。

例 14: It will be interesting to see how the story of microbiota and inflammation in the pathogenesis of depression unfolds. With technology and social structures mutating faster than ever, measuring and monitoring the effects of these hyperbolic changes on mental health will be important.

观察微生物群和炎症在抑郁症发病机制中如何开展,就会非常有趣。随着技术和社会结构的变化比以往任何时候都要快,测量和监测这些双曲线变化对心理健康的影响将非常重要。

第四节　练习巩固

1. 将括号中的中文译成英语。

(1) Additionally, an ideal fabric that minimizes bacterial colonization has not been identified; in fact, ＿＿＿＿＿＿＿＿＿(迄今为止研究结果互相矛盾). More robust research, ＿＿＿＿＿＿＿＿＿＿＿＿＿(最好是对照实验), needs to be conducted to determine the binding potential and length of survival of microbes on various fabrics.

(2) In general, the findings of this review are ＿＿＿＿＿＿＿＿(与其他综述大体一致), all of which reported that a chlorhexidine solution was better than a povidone solution for CVC care. However, ＿＿＿＿＿＿＿＿(我们不能确定) whether each disinfectant was combined with alcohol or an aqueous solution, the latter of which was found to be better. ＿＿＿＿＿＿＿＿＿＿＿＿＿＿＿(我们需要更多的证据).

（3）Extended hospital stays may _____（进一步增加医院感染和不良事件的风险）. In fact，a 6% incremental daily risk of experiencing an adverse event has been previously reported for each day of hospital admission.

（4）_____（数据表明）that colonization by MDROs is associated with higher rates of infection and outbreaks in clinical settings. _____（这对医护人员有重要影响），especially those who routinely care for immunocompromised or intensive care unit patients.

（5）_____（正如我们的分析以及尼日利亚和美国输入的埃博拉病毒病例所显示的那样），the potential for further international spread via air travel remains present.

2. 请将下面句子翻译成英语。

（1）采用小剂量 CT 筛查可以降低肺癌导致的死亡率。

_____

（2）严重低血糖症与一系列不良临床转归的危险性上升有关。

_____

（3）在非洲这些资源有限的环境中，液体推注（fluid boluses）显著增加了有灌注受损（impaired perfusion）危重患儿的 48 小时死亡率。

_____

（4）特定的饮食和生活方式因素与长期体重增加独立相关，对预防肥胖的策略有显著的总效应（aggregate effect）和影响。

_____

（5）与美国普通人群一样，活体肾脏提供者中存在医疗条件的种族差异。

_____

3. 阅读下列论文中的讨论节选部分，并分析其语言特征。

Discussion

Our study shows that many investigators have documented bacterial colonization of hospital attire. It is important to note，however，that a direct relationship between bacterial contamination of HCW's clothing and hospital-acquired infection has，to our knowledge，not been demonstrated. In fact，some experts argue that there is little to implicate an association between the two. Hambraeus has demonstrated that bacteria can be transferred from nursing gowns to both patients and bed linens. However，there is no definitive evidence that has linked bacterial colonization of attire with health care-associated infections（HAIs）. One sole exception to this is a case series conducted by Barrie et al，in which 2 patients were diagnosed with Bacillus cereus meningitis status postneurosurgery. An investigation concluded that lint from bed linens contaminated with B cereus spores likely served as the transmission source, eventually resulting in wound infection.

Strategies to reduce bacterial contamination of white coats include sanitizing sleeves and pockets regularly in addition to altering the coat itself by shortening the overall length and sleeves. In 2007, the UK Department of Health implemented BBE, a dress code requiring HCWs to wear attire with short sleeves or rolled up sleeves, and no white coats, jewelry, ties, watches, or rings when seeing patients at the bedside, to decrease nosocomial infections. This initiative was associated with a decrease in HAIs over a 5-year period, from 8.2% in 2006 to 6.4% in 2011. The policy is also now reflected in UK legislation. Presumably, BBE allows for maintenance of proper hand hygiene, which has proven to be cost-effective in the reduction of nosocomial infections. Bearman et al reviewed hospital policies regarding HCW attire of 7 US institutions, finding that each outlined generic dress code requirements specifying professional attire, but did not address specifics aside from operating room attire (scrubs, masks, head covers, and footwear). Only 1 institution provided recommendations for physicians, and that was the BBE policy. Widespread adoption of similar provider attire policies may be beneficial for countries such as the United States.

The use of proprietary antimicrobial coating on scrubs has increased in the last decade to combat colonization of bacteria on textiles. However, conclusions from several studies in this systematic review reveal no statistically significant differences between standard scrubs and scrubs treated with antimicrobial coating. The possibility remains that these studies may be underpowered.

Effectively reducing the spread of nosocomial infections and MDROs requires effort both by providers and hospital systems, starting with awareness of safe hygiene practices. Duroy and Le Coutour surveyed medical students in clinical rotations, finding that 66.5% of students were dissatisfied by the quality of hospital hygiene training. Almost half reported being unaware of differences between antiseptic and simple handwashing practices. Munoz-Price et al found a statistically significant association between contamination of hands and white coats. Notably, this association was not observed with hands and scrubs, possibly owing to increased frequency of laundering. These findings support a call for action for quality and safety committees to improve hygiene curriculum and provider attire guidelines. Suggestions for HCWs and hospitals are included in Table 4.

This systematic review is not without limitations. Each study provides its own set of guidance based on author opinion/rationale, practical considerations, and evidence of relatively low power. Differences also existed in methodology for culturing and sampling attire with studies searching for and targeting a variable set of isolates. There remains need for more robust research regarding potentially pathogenic bacterial transmission through HCW attire. Moreover, the efficacy of industrial versus domestic laundering of attire remains unexplored on a large scale, with research implicating the dilution of water, water temperature, and bleach level as potential factors in post-laundering microbial contamination of HCW attire.

A distinction must be made between bacterial colonization and infection. Pathogens such as S aureus are often colonized in nasal epithelium, skin, hair, and other locations of healthy individuals. Clinically, however, it is the possibility of infection that is critical—that is, when these contaminants result in activation of pathological processes. Ascertaining the quantitative risk of spread of direct infection from HCW attire is challenging given real-world constraints and difficulty in mitigating confounding factors, even in controlled studies. Data reveal that colonization by MDROs is associated with higher rates of infection and outbreaks in clinical settings. This has important implications for providers, especially those who routinely care for immunocompromised or intensive care unit patients. Although there is no definitive evidence that HCW attire directly contributes to HAIs, the evidence that increased colonization can serve as a silent reservoir that causes infection in high-risk groups is compelling.

CONCLUSIONS

Hospitals worldwide are concerned about infection control and have implemented numerous patient safety protocols to combat horizontal transmission of infectious agents. The findings of this review suggest that provider attire is a potential source of transmission for pathogenic bacteria in health care settings. However, data confirming a direct link between provider attire and HAIs remains limited. It seems appropriate to develop protocols needed to reduce contamination of both white coats and surgical scrubs. The suggestions outlined in this article, based on available evidence, may serve as a guideline for health care professionals and hospital systems to reduce the spread of bacterial pathogens, including MDROs, that have the potential to precipitate hospital-acquired infections.

第八章　病例报告

第一节　病例报告的内容

1.1　定义

病例报告(case reports)是医学论文的一种常见体裁。不同于入院大病历、病程记录和病例讨论等,病例报告通过对某些特殊的病例进行详细的科学观察、记录和描述,试图在疾病的临床表现、发病机制、实验室检查、影像学检查、诊断、治疗及预防等方面提供第一手的资料。

1.2　病例报告的内容特点

(1) 首次发现的病例,比如艾滋病、新冠肺炎等;
(2) 疾病有特殊的临床表现、影像学及检验学等手段的新发现、特殊的临床转归、诊断和治疗过程中的特殊经验和教训;
(3) 临床少见、报道较少、难以诊断的罕见病例。

1.3　病例报告的写作要求

英文病例报告的写作要求比较严格。病例报告中要求提供新信息,强调尊重患者的隐私,很多期刊要求提供患者签字的知情同意书,病例报告可包含单个或多个病例,长度为1 000—2 500字,参考文献10—30篇。不同期刊有不同要求,比如《新英格兰医学杂志》(*The New England Journal of Medicine*)将病例报告分为 Brief Report 和 Clinical Problem Solving 两种,前者要求字数不超过2 000字,摘要部分字数不超过100字,表格和图片不超过3个,参考文献不超过25篇;而后者则要求字数在2 500以内,参考文献为15篇以内。

1.4　病例报告的结构

不同的期刊对病例报告的写作形式要求不尽相同,一般来说病例报告由以下部分构成：

    （1）题目（Title）

    （2）作者（Author）

    （3）摘要（Abstract）

    （4）前言（Introduction）

    （5）病例描述（Case Description）

    （6）讨论（Discussion）

    （7）结论（Conclusion）

    （8）参考文献（References）

有些期刊的格式较为特殊，比如《柳叶刀》（Lancet）杂志，它不包含摘要和前言，而是病例介绍和讨论融在一起；还有一些期刊要求按照一般文章的格式，即摘要、前言、方法、结果、讨论、参考文献来撰写。

第二节　病例报告范例分析

下面我们挑选病例报告的几个主要构成部分，具体分析几篇病例报告的语言特点。

2.1　摘要

摘要（Abstract）是整个病例的简介，分结构性和非结构性两种，字数一般为 150 字以内。注意，不是所有的病例报告都要求写摘要。

例 1：非结构性摘要

Abstract：Acute phlegmonous gastritis（APG）is an extremely uncommon and potentially rapid fatal systemic infection with very few reported cases in the literature. This case report demonstrates a case of idiopathic APG in an afebrile, otherwise healthy individual that resolved with broad-spectrum antibiotic therapy and did not require operative management.

【分析】

这是《美国急诊医学会杂志》（*Journal of the American College of Emergency Physicians*）上刊登的一篇关于急性痰性胃炎病例报告的摘要部分，是一篇非结构性摘要，主要介绍了该病例的基本信息。

【实用表达】

    • ... is an extremely uncommon ... 非常罕见

    • ... with very few reported cases in the literature 在文献中报道的病例很少

【句型模仿】

• This case report demonstrates a case of ...

该病例报告展示了一个……的病例

【长难句理解】

• This case report demonstrates a case of idiopathic APG in an afebrile, otherwise healthy individual that resolved with broad-spectrum antibiotic therapy and did not require operative management.

这句话较长,是一个复合句,主干为主谓宾结构,主语为"This case report",谓语是"demonstrates",宾语为名词"case",其后带有介词短语构成的定语"of idiopathic APG in an afebrile, otherwise healthy individual"。需要注意此介词短语中的名词individual又带有that引导的定语从句,表述此患者接受的治疗。

此病例报告展示了一例特发性急性痰性胃炎(APG)患者,不发烧,无其他不适,接受广谱抗生素治疗后症状消退而不需要进行手术。

例 2:结构性摘要

Background

There are thousands of survivors of the 2014 Ebola outbreak in west Africa. Ebola virus can persist in survivors for months in immune-privileged sites; however, viral relapse causing life-threatening and potentially transmissible disease has not been described. We report a case of late relapse in a patient who had been treated for severe Ebola virus disease with high viral load (peak cycle threshold value 13.2).

Methods

A 39-year-old female nurse from Scotland, who had assisted the humanitarian effort in Sierra Leone, had received intensive supportive treatment and experimental antiviral therapies, and had been discharged with undetectable Ebola virus RNA in peripheral blood. The patient was readmitted to hospital 9 months after discharge with symptoms of acute meningitis, and was found to have Ebola virus in cerebrospinal fluid (CSF). She was treated with supportive therapy and experimental antiviral drug GS-5734 (Gilead Sciences, San Francisco, Foster City, CA, USA). We monitored Ebola virus RNA in CSF and plasma, and sequenced the viral genome using an unbiased metagenomic approach.

Findings

On admission, reverse transcriptase PCR identified Ebola virus RNA at a higher level in CSF (cycle threshold value 23.7) than plasma (31.3); infectious virus was only recovered from CSF. The patient developed progressive meningoencephalitis with cranial neuropathies and radiculopathy. Clinical recovery was associated with addition of high-dose corticosteroids during GS-5734 treatment. CSF Ebola virus

RNA slowly declined and was undetectable following 14 days of treatment with GS-5734. Sequencing of plasma and CSF viral genome revealed only two noncoding changes compared with the original infecting virus.

Interpretation

Our report shows that previously unanticipated，late，severe relapses of Ebola virus can occur，in this case in the CNS. This finding fundamentally redefines what is known about the natural history of Ebola virus infection. Vigilance should be maintained in the thousands of Ebola survivors for cases of relapsed infection. The potential for these cases to initiate new transmission chains is a serious public health concern.

【分析】

这是《柳叶刀》杂志上一篇有关埃博拉病毒复发导致脑膜脑炎的病例报告的摘要部分。这是一篇结构性摘要，由背景、方法、发现、评述四个部分构成。第 1 段介绍埃博拉病毒的特点及研究现状中的不足。第 2 段描述一个病例的相关病史，接受过的检测和干预措施。第 3 段比较患者入院时以及进行抗病毒治疗后的一些临床指针，揭示病毒复发与原始病毒感染相比存在的变化。第 4 段从本研究的结果出发强调它的指导意义，即埃博拉病毒的复发提醒人们应保持对此类病例的警惕。

【实用表达】

- viral relapse 病毒复发
- immune-privileged sites 免疫赦免区
- high viral load 高病毒载量
- life-threatening and potentially transmissible disease 危及生命和具有潜在传染性的疾病
- intensive supportive treatment 强化支持治疗
- experimental antiviral therapies 实验性抗病毒疗法
- be discharged 出院
- be readmitted to 再次入院
- on admission 入院时

【句型模仿】

1. This finding fundamentally redefines what is known about ...
这一发现从根本上重新定义了我们对于……的已知内容

2. Vigilance should be maintained in ...
我们应该保持对……的警惕

3. The potential for ... is a serious public health concern
潜在的……是一个严重的公共卫生问题

【长难句理解】

1. A 39-year-old female nurse from Scotland, who had assisted the humanitarian effort in Sierra Leone, had received intensive supportive treatment and experimental antiviral therapies, and had been discharged with undetectable Ebola virus RNA in peripheral blood.

这是一个典型的复合句,who 引导的非限制定语从句中的谓语成分较多导致句子偏长,谓语动词有 had assisted、had received 和 had been discharged,均为过去完成时态,介绍患者在疾病复发前的一些基本情况,包括接受的治疗和出院前的情况。值得注意的是,此处使用一个复合句比三个单句更适合表达科技文体中凝练的意思。此句大意为:患者为一名 39 岁苏格兰女护士,曾协助塞拉利昂的人道主义工作,接受过强化支持治疗和实验性抗病毒治疗,出院时外周血检测不到病毒 RNA。

2. Clinical recovery was associated with addition of high-dose corticosteroids during GS-5734 treatment. CSF Ebola virus RNA slowly declined and was undetectable following 14 days of treatment with GS-5734.

这两句是对患者治疗结果的表述,第一句中的短语 be associated with 表示原因,用在此处非常地道。第二句中注意表示数值变化的英文表达,slowly declined "缓慢下降",undetectable "直至消失",这是一个用词缀法构成的单词,在科技文献中很常见。此句大意为:在 GS-5734 治疗期间添加高剂量皮质类固醇促进恢复。脑脊液埃博拉病毒 RNA 缓慢下降,在使用 GS-5734 治疗 14 天后无法检测到。

2.2 前言

前言(Introduction)给出病例的背景,阐明病例的相关性和重要性,必要处给出相关文献。和综述相似,前言对全篇有引导作用。注意,不是所有的病例报告都要求有前言。

例 3:Malignant melanoma occurs most frequently in skin but also in many organs and tissues of the body. However, primary hepatic malignant melanoma is exceedingly rare. Only 12 cases, including 8 cases from PubMed and 4 cases from Chinese literature, have been reported. In PubMed, there are only 3 cases of definite primary melanoma. Microscopically, it may be easily misdiagnosed because of morphological heterogeneity and hypomelanotic appearance. The present case represents the only case encountered in our department. In this report, we describe our pathological observations and review the literature in order to improve our understanding of this disease, avoid misdiagnosis and provide evidence for its clinical treatment and prognosis.

【分析】

这是一篇介绍原发性肝恶性黑色素瘤病例报告的前言部分,内容简短,首先指出病例罕见,且容易误诊,表明此病例为作者所在医院第一例,最后一句话指出描述病理特点的目的是为避免误诊,为临床诊断提供依据。

【实用表达】

- ... is exceedingly rare ……是极为罕见的
- ... may be easily misdiagnosed ……极易误诊

【句型模仿】

1. The present case represents the only case encountered in our department.

本病例是我们科室遇到的唯一病例。

2. We describe our pathological observations and review the literature in order to improve our understanding of this disease, avoid misdiagnosis and provide evidence for its clinical treatment and prognosis.

在本报告中,我们描述了我们的病理观察并回顾了文献,以提高我们对该疾病的理解,避免误诊,并为其临床治疗和预后提供证据。

【参考译文】

恶性黑色素瘤最常发生在皮肤上,但也发生在身体的许多器官和组织中。然而,原发性肝恶性黑色素瘤却极为罕见。仅报道12例,其中PubMed 8例,中国文献4例。在PubMed中,只有3例明确为原发性黑色素瘤。由于形态异质性和低黑素外观,此病在镜下容易误诊。本病例是我们科室遇到的唯一病例。在本报告中,我们描述了我们的病理观察并回顾了文献,以提高我们对该疾病的理解,避免误诊,并为其临床治疗和预后提供证据。

2.3 病例描述

病例描述(Case Description)提供病例详细信息,内容较多,可以参照住院病历,按临床诊疗的常规顺序进行写作,常用时态为一般过去时。具体内容包括:患者基本信息(Patient description)、现病史(Case history)、体格检查(Physical examination results)、辅助检查(Results of pathological tests and other investigations)、诊疗计划(Treatment plan)、预期结果(Expected outcome of the treatment plan)、实际结果(Actual outcome)。注意,病例描述不能完全照搬住院病历,需要提供影像学检查、仪器设备等图片,进行临床量表评定的数据表,还要特别注意保护患者隐私,很多英文期刊都要求提交知情同意书(Informed consent)。

例4:An 84-year-old male patient had a mass in his right axilla for more than 20 years. He came for further treatment due to its progressive growth for 11 months with bloody ulceration for more than 1 month. The initial size of the mass was 1.0 cm × 1.5 cm × 1.0 cm, similar to the size of a piece of peanut. It was hard and immovable. The boundary between tumor and normal skin was unclear. About 11 months ago, the patient felt the mass was increasing rapidly, expanding to 2. 5 cm ×2. 4 cm×1. 8 cm in size, and raised 1. 0 cm above the skin surface (Fig. 1). Besides, the pain when touched gradually became conspicuous. One month ago, the mass started to swell and ulcerate. No signs of enlargement of bilateral supraclavicular lymph nodes were found.

Auxiliary examination:

1. Positron emission computed tomography showed the following:

(1) A nodule of the density of subcutaneous soft tissue in the right axilla, the boundary was unclear, some layers protruded to the skin surface, with increase of metabolism. The Standardized Uptake Value max level was 8. 8, considered malignant tumor.

(2) Two enlarged lymph nodes in the right axilla, with abnormal increase of metabolism. The Standardized Uptake Value max level was 13. 0, considered lymph node metastasis.

(3) No significant signs of malignant primary tumor in other parts of the body.

2. Pathological Test: Grade Ⅱ infiltrating ductal carcinoma derived from the accessory mammary gland (right axilla) with invasion of local skin.

3. Immunohistochemical examination result: estrogen receptor (＋＋) 90%, progesterone receptor (＋＋＋) 100%, human epidermal growth factor receptor-2 (1＋), ki67 (20% positive), prostate specific antigen (－), caudal-related homeobox-2 (－), thyroid transcription factor-1 (－), synaptophysin (＋), NapsinA (1), and CK7 (－) (Figs. 2 and 3).

After exclusion of operative contraindications, we decided to perform radical mastectomy of the accessory mammary gland and adjacent lymph nodes clearance under general anesthesia. First, we performed a spindle-shaped incision which was 3. 0 cm around the mass. Second, the accessory mammary gland and the spindle-shaped skin flap were integrally dissociated by electronic knife. Thirdly, interpectoral lymph nodes, lateral pectoralis minor lymph nodes, anterior latissimus dorsi lymph nodes, axillary lymph nodes, posterior pectoralis minor lymph nodes were removed successively. Then, we removed the specimen after ligating and cutting off the arteries, veins and lymph glands. During the operation, we protected long thoracic nerve and dorsal thoracic vascular nerve. The operational region was irrigated with warm water (36 ℃ - 37 ℃), and the bleeding was arrested thoroughly. Parasternal and axillary drainage tubes were placed respectively. Finally, the operational region was packed with pressure bandage for at least 5 days (Figs. 4 and 5).

According to the Guidelines of Treatments for Breast Diseases in 2017, we decided to provide this patient with only endocrine therapy postoperatively. We recommended that the patient should take Letrozole orally for the rest of his life. The patient recovered uneventfully and was discharged 3 days postoperatively, with no significant pain, hematoma, infection, or any functional disorder during upper limb activities. The patient was followed up regularly every 3 to 6 months, and no signs of recurrence were observed.

【分析】

这是一篇关于男性腋窝副乳腺癌病例报告的病例描述部分,由四段构成,时态为一般过去时。第1段是患者的基本资料,包括性别、年龄、一般特征、主诉。第2段提供体格检查和实验室检查结果,包括CT扫描、病理检查及免疫组化的结果。第3段是诊疗过程,描述了在全身麻醉下进行副乳腺根治性乳房切除术及邻近淋巴结清扫术。第4段是有关术后用药、预后和随访的内容。可以看出,病例描述部分基本可以按照住院大病历的内容来写。但是需要注意的是,切忌将原始病历照搬,可以省略其中不重要的内容,避免使用各种非客观性,各种怀疑或推测性语句。

【实用表达】

• The patient came for further treatment due to ... 患者由于……来接受进一步治疗

• The initial size of the mass was ... 肿块的初始大小是……

• The boundary between ... and ... was unclear ……和……边界不清

• exclusion of operative contraindications 排除手术禁忌征

• perform ... under general anesthesia 在全身麻醉下进行……手术

【句型模仿】

病例描述部分根据病例的不同,所用表达也不尽相同,但是仍然有些常见的句型可供参考,具体如下。

1. 描述病状和体征的常见句型

• A man aged 50 was admitted for/with ... 男性患者,50岁,因……入院

• The temperature peaked/dropped to ... 体温升至/降至……

• His conditions were deteriorated/aggravated thereafter. 他的病情很快恶化/加重。

• The patient was referred by his family physician to our out-patient clinic, complaining of ... 患者由家庭医生转诊至我院门诊,主诉……

2. 描述体检结果的常见句型

• No abnormality was found on the liver. 肝未见异常。

• Laparoscopy showed/revealed abnormal changes. 腹腔镜检查显示异常改变。

• The general gynecological examination was unremarkable/insignificant. 妇科常规检查未发现明显异常。

• A mass was detected/noted. 检查出/显示有肿块。

3. 描述诊断和治疗的常见表达

• She was diagnosed with/suffering ... 她被诊断患有……

• ... was given the diagnosis of ... 被诊断为……

• We recommended that the patient should take Letrozole orally for the rest of his life. 我们建议患者在余生中口服来曲唑。

• The patient was subjected to the implantation of cardiac pacemakers. 患者被植入心脏起搏器。

• The patient tolerated the operative procedure quite well. 该病人手术过程耐受良好。

4. 描述原因的常见表达

• ... may be due to ... 可能由……所致

• ... may be responsible/accountable for ... ……可能导致/引起……的原因

• This is one factor that may induce/cause/lead to/bring about ... 该因素可能成为导致……的一个原因

5. 描述进展和预后的常见表达

• The patient recovered uneventfully and was discharged 3 days postoperatively, with no significant pain, hematoma, infection, or any functional disorder.

患者顺利恢复,术后 3 天出院,无明显疼痛、血肿、感染或任何功能障碍。

• The patient was followed up regularly every 3 to 6 months, no signs of recurrence were observed.

患者每 3—6 个月定期随访一次,未见复发迹象。

• Clinical improvement can be expected within a week, but full recovery may take one month at least.

病情一周内有望改善,但痊愈至少需要一个月。

• The general conditions of the patient indicate a poor/promising outlook.

该病人的一般情况表明预后不佳/良好。

注意,关于预后的描述有的也可以用一般现在时态。

【长难句理解】

• The patient recovered uneventfully and was discharged 3 days postoperatively, with no significant pain, hematoma, infection, or any functional disorder during upper limb activities. The patient was followed up regularly every 3 to 6 months, no signs of recurrence were observed.

此为病例描述中对病例的实际结果和随访情况的说明。此句大意为:患者顺利康复,术后 3 天出院,上肢活动时无明显疼痛、血肿、感染或任何功能紊乱。患者每 3 至 6 个月定期随访一次,未观察到复发迹象。

2.4 讨论

讨论(Discussion)部分非常重要,往往决定着能否说服编辑接收整篇病例报告。它是前言内容的扩展,具体包括:描述疾病背景、总结本病例的发现、展开说明本病例的特点,有时需要列举文献与其他研究或病例对比,有时还包括部分结论的内容,即病例的处理经验、教训和意义。

例5:We experienced a rare case of the patient who had both EGFR mutation and EML4-ALK fusion gene. To the best of our knowledge, five patients with both mutations have been reported so far in the world. Four patients received EGFR-TKI therapy (Table 1). Two cases showed good response, whereas the other two cases did not. We report the 5th case which also did not show good response. In general, the response rate to EGFR-TKI therapy in the patients with EGFR mutation is 70%—80%, however, these 5 cases with both mutations tend to be less responsive. In the preclinical study, EML4-ALK positive NSCLC was not responsive to erlotinib therapy. EGFR TKI therapy showed no effects to the all 10 patients with EML4-ALK fusion gene, although, there were no patients harboring both EGFR mutation and EML4-ALK in these papers. Whereas, EML4-ALK positive patients had a longer progression free survival after PEM therapy compared with EGFR mutant patients.

In our case, the characteristics of the patient were young age, light-smoker and acinar pattern adenocaricinoma which showed similarity with the ones of EML4-ALK positive NSCLC. Additionally, PEM therapy showed a good response to our patient, whereas erlotinib therapy did not. In the cases with these both mutations, EML4-ALK gene may play a main role in the oncogenesis for some unknown reasons. Although ALK inhibitor was effective to EML4-ALK positive NSCLC, it was not on the market in Japan at that point. Further experience and the understanding of the lung cancer molecular biology are required for the better treatment of the cases with both EGFR mutation and EML4-ALK fusion gene.

【分析】

这是一篇有关肺腺癌突变的病例报告的讨论部分。1—3句介绍背景和本病例的发现。4—7句列举文献。最后一段主要介绍了 EGFR 和 EML4-ALK 基因在肺腺癌中发生了共同突变,在临床上比较少见。

【实用表达】

• We experienced a rare case of the patient who ... 一例……罕见病例

• To the best of our knowledge,... have been reported so far in the world. 据我们所知,到目前为止世界上已经有……患者被报道过。

- In the preclinical study, ... was not responsive to ... 在临床前研究中, ……对……治疗无反应。

- In our case, the characteristics of the patient were ... 在我们的病例中,患者的特征是……

- Additionally, ... therapy showed a good response to our patient, whereas ... therapy did not. 此外,……治疗对我们的患者有良好的反应,而……治疗则没有。

- ... may play a main role in the oncogenesis for some unknown reasons ……可能在肿瘤发生过程中起主要作用,原因不明

- further experience and the understanding of ... are required for the better treatment of the cases with ... 为了更好地治疗……的病例,需要……更多的经验和理解

【句型模仿】

讨论部分常用来给出结论,或者提出警告和强调重要性。一般常见句型如下:

- In conclusion/To sum up/Therefore, an ophthalmic opinion is warranted when facial pain is associated with visual symptoms of features or ocular inflammation.

总之,如果面部疼痛与视觉症状或眼炎有联系,就有理由断定为眼病。

- One lesson of this case is the necessity for a detailed history before intervention.

从该病例中所得到的启发是干预前需要详细询问病史。

- It is important to emphasize that the necessary long and extensive surgery carries a higher risk of infection with a substantial risk of death.

应当强调的是时间长、手术大的手术让患者发生感染的风险更高,甚至存在死亡的风险。

【长难句理解】

- In general, the response rate to EGFR-TKI therapy in the patients with EGFR mutation is 70%—80%, however, these 5 cases with both mutations tend to be less responsive. In the preclinical study, EML4-ALK positive NSCLC was not responsive to erlotinib therapy. EGFR TKI therapy showed no effects to the all 10 patients with EML4-ALK fusion gene, although, there were no patients harboring both EGFR mutation and EML4-ALK in these papers. Whereas, EML4-ALK positive patients had a longer progression free survival after PEM therapy compared with EGFR mutant patients.

这三句是病例讨论的中间部分,将文献中报道的肺腺癌病例与本病例进行对比,指出两种基因在肺腺癌中发生共同突变的情况比较少见,传统治疗的效果有限,需要寻求新的治疗方法。值得注意的是,句意中上下文转折意思较多,作者运用了三个不同的转

折词进行同义替换,即 however、although、whereas。此句大意为:

一般来说,EGFR 突变患者对 EGFR-TKI 治疗的有效率为 70%—80%,然而这 5 例同时存在两种突变的患者往往反应较差。在临床前研究中,EML4-ALK 阳性的 NSCLC 对埃洛替尼治疗没有反应。EGFR-TKI 治疗对所有 10 名携带 EML4-ALK 融合基因的患者均无影响,尽管在这些论文中没有报道同时携带 EGFR 突变和 EML4-ALK 的患者。然而,与 EGFR 突变患者相比,EML4-ALK 阳性患者在 PEM 治疗后的无进展生存期更长。

2.5 结论

结论(Conclusion)部分是对病例的总结和建议,需要给出临床处理的经验教训等。有的病例报告在讨论部分的最后一两句或者最后一段就描述了结论的内容。此部分一般回答两个问题:下次遇到同样的情况如何应对? 给临床和科研提供了怎样的建议? 内容简明扼要,1—2 句话即可。结论部分主要使用一般现在时态。

例 6:We report a rare case of lung cancer harboring both EGFR mutation and EML4-ALK fusion gene. PEM therapy showed a good response to the patient, whereas erlotinib therapy did not. Oncologists should be aware of the possibility of the multiple mutations.

【分析】
这是上例病例报告中的结论部分,指出报告的内容、临床上要注意的方面,主要是总结和建议。

【参考译文】
我们对一个罕见的肺癌病例做了报告,该患者同时携带 EGFR 突变和 EML4-ALK 融合基因。PEM 治疗对患者反应良好,而厄洛替尼治疗则没有。肿瘤学家应该意识到多重突变的可能性。

第三节 练习巩固

1. 阅读下列病例报告的前言部分,试将其翻译成汉语,并体会其中的语言特征。

This case report describes an elderly female with features of cognitive decline and depression, living at home alone, who was referred to our social care service after diagnosis of Alzheimer's disease. Depression is a risk factor for, and common neuropsychiatric symptom of, dementia. Both dementia and depression can result in cognitive and functional impairment and deterioration in quality of life. Social isolation is a both risk factor for, as well as potential consequence of dementia and depression.

With high levels of undetected dementia and depression in older people in China, where specialized dementia social care services remain rare, there is a need for practical, symptom-focused solutions to delivering dementia care in the community. Our dementia social care delivery team has developed a novel, community-based, multicomponent, non-pharmacological intervention program for the management of people with Alzheimer's disease and dementia.

2. 请将括号里的中文翻译成英语。

Primary hepatic malignant melanoma is a very rare disease. 1) _____
_____（为了提供诊断、鉴别诊断和发病机制的线索），
a case of a 49 year-old female patient with primary hepatic malignant melanoma is presented. B-mode ultrasound and contrast-enhanced abdominal computerized tomography (CT) examinations revealed that 2) _____
_____（增大的肝脏中弥漫分布着大小不等的结节）.
Pathological examination revealed that tumor cells with poor differentiation were located in nests with prominent melanin deposition. Immuno-histochemical staining showed that the tumor cells were positive for HMB-45 and S-100 protein. 3) _____
_____（未发现其他部位的原发
性黑色素瘤的证据） by comprehensive examinations. Therefore, the patient was diagnosed with primary malignant melanoma of liver. Our case showed that primary malignant melanoma of liver is of histological heterogeneity, and immunohisto-chemical staining 4) _____
［有助于其与其他肝脏肿瘤（hepatic neoplasms）的鉴别诊断］。

3. 下列句子选自一篇病例报告的讨论部分，但顺序排列错误，请将下列句子重新排序，并分析每个句子的功能。

1. Our patient with advanced breast cancer had severe cachexia.

2. Consequently, a vicious cycle occurs, with malnutrition from insufficient dietary intake resulting in increasing therapy toxicity and the unmanaged tumor causing even more severe malnutrition.

3. Although cancer-related cachexia is often attributed to loss of appetite and the side effects of chemotherapy, it may be closely associated with the destruction of normal tissue by tumor secretory factors and clinical events or therapeutic interventions.

4. The mechanism by which cachexia promotes tumor invasion and metastasis is not yet clear, but it may be related to the inflammatory response, hypoxic state, decreased leptin levels and release of pro-angiogenic factors in cachexia patients.

5. As we focus on weight loss, we attempt to define cachexia more comprehensively through body composition, to be incorporated into routine clinical practice.

第九章　医学综述

　　医学综述（Medical review）简称综述，是指对某一医学专题文献材料进行收集、整理、分析、归纳和比较之后撰写的综合、总结和评论性文章，属于二次文献资料。医学综述是医学论文的重要文体之一，很多医学期刊都有特设的综述专栏。综述的作者通常是期刊特别邀请的、对某个专业有着较深了解和研究的专家。

　　综述性文章和原创文章的区别在于，综述性文章更为专门全面、深入系统地论述某一研究领域的问题，对所综述的内容进行综合、分析、评价，反映作者的观点和见解，并与综述的内容构成整体。文献综述之所以具有指导性，是因为它能对研究问题进行定义和分类，总结前人的研究成果以便让读者了解当前的研究现状，找出文献的相关性、矛盾性，并提出解决问题的方法和建议。通过阅读综述和参考文献，后来的研究者们可在较短的时间里获得较多关于某个研究领域系统、具体的信息，掌握该领域研究进展和发展方向，从而选择新的研究目标与突破点。

　　按照时间的不同，医学文献综述可分为回顾性综述（Retrospective review）和前瞻性综述（Prospective review）。按照作者论述方式的不同，医学文献综述可分为归纳性综述（Deductive review）和评论性综述（Critical review）。按照具体内容的不同，医学文献综述可分为动态性综述（Developmental review）、成就性综述（Result review）和争鸣性综述（Contentious review）。

　　目前最常见的医学文献综述按结构类型分成叙述性综述（Narrative review）和系统性综述（Systematic review）。由于目标读者、研究性质、纳入标准等方面固有的差异，两类综述各自呈现出一些语言特点。叙述性综述的结构框架相对松散，文中小节标题的使用较为自由，过渡语和连接词的使用较多，以维持文本的连贯；而系统性综述结构固定，小节标题的使用一般严格遵守前言、方法、结果和讨论（IMRAD）格式，技术路线图和数据表格更多，将正文主干切割成更多语义独立的小板块，因此，除文字较多且文本连贯性较强的结果部分，并不太倚重连接词。

　　医学文献综述的本质特点决定了其写作的基本规范。下面就叙述性综述和系统性综述的写作内容和格式进行探讨。

第一节 叙述性综述

叙述性综述(Narrative review)是根据特定的目标和需要,收集有关文献资料,采用定性分析的方法,对论文中阐述的研究目的、方法、结果、结论和观点进行分析和评价。

叙述性综述并无固定格式,通常和原创文章一样包括摘要(Abstract)、前言(Introduction)、主体部分(Main body)或结论(Summary\Conclusion)几个部分。

1.1 摘要

一般来说,叙述性综述有或没有摘要部分都可以。如期刊要求提供的话,要选取和内容最为相关的要点,一般不超过200词,同时附上至少三个关键词。

1.2 前言

和原创文章一样,作者在前言部分提出问题,进行定义性解释或介绍研究背景等,常用一般现在时或现在完成时;陈述文献综述的目的和内容时,常用一般现在时或一般将来时。

1.3 主体部分

文章的主体部分可因文章字数、内容、所涉及的范围及作者的写作技巧有所不同。常用方法:(1)按选题所属学科的内在科学规律分层阐述,遵循该学科的常规思维程序及逻辑原则;(2)按目前争论的焦点分别提出问题加以论述;(3)按学科进展分阶段论述(时间顺序),或按既有发现或理论的重要性排序;(4)按临床诊疗工作程序分述等。

例:在一篇题目为"Depression as a disease of modernity: Explanations for increasing prevalence"的综述论文的目录可以看到该文章的写作框架。

Contents

1. Introduction

2. An epidemic of depression

3. Possible explanations for changing rates

4. Key environmental changes

4.1. Obesity

4.2. Diet

4.3. Physical activity

4.4. Light and sleep

4.5. Social environment

5. Future directions and implications

作者在主体的前言部分(Introduction)提出并解释了现代性疾病(disease of modernity)的概念和文中所讨论的抑郁症(depression)的含义,以及两者之间的假设关系。作者指出,虽然现有数据表明年轻群体的抑郁症患病率在上升,终生患病的风险也在增加,但由于现有文献结果相互矛盾,研究方法存在缺陷,目前尚未得出有力的结论。于是作者在前言的最后提出本综述探讨的两个基本问题:① 抑郁症发病率是否有所上升? ② 如果是,原因是什么?

在第二部分(An epidemic of depression),文章综述了抑郁症在流行病学科领域的研究发展历程。作者认为,只针对临床人群测量(而非社区抽样)、回顾性研究的回忆偏差以及纵向调查的结果不一致等问题困扰着对抑郁症的研究。同时指出,流行病学的纵向研究大多证实了抑郁症发病率在上升。

在第三部分(Possible explanations for changing rates),作者给出了导致抑郁症发病率上升的可能解释,接着在第四部分(Key environmental changes)重点讨论了外界环境因素的影响,比如肥胖、节食、缺乏体育锻炼等。综述最后的第五部分(Future directions and implications),作者呼吁未来开展更多抑郁症相关研究,并需要采取的政策干预,以应对这一公共健康危机。这篇综述的主体部分基本按照前面方法(1)的思路来写作的。

不论采用何种写作方法,主体内容应着重论述所研究专题的历史与现状、发展趋势、各学派的主要观点和依据、争论的焦点、当前研究的新发现和主要问题、存在的薄弱环节和对未来发展前景的展望等。

1.4　结论

叙述性综述的结论部分和原创论文一样要讨论文章的局限性及临床意义,且要附有大量的参考文献。

由于叙述性综述研究的问题相对宽泛,对原始文献的检索和分析也不如系统性综述严密,定性分析多于定量分析,因此使用上不如系统性综述普遍。鉴于目前国际上许多综述类医学期刊只接受约稿专家撰写的叙述性综述,例如像 *JRM* (Journal of Rehabilitation Medicine) 这样专门发表综述性文章的期刊,在 "Information for Authors" 中这么描述:

"However, *JRM*, as many other journals, is reluctant to publish narrative reviews unless there is a compelling reason for doing so. You should therefore always consult the Editor-in-Chief before submitting such a manuscript. *Journal of Rehabilitation Medicine* has a restrictive policy regarding publication of narrative reviews. "

因此在投寄叙述性综述的稿件前一定要咨询期刊编辑室。

第二节 系统性综述

系统性综述（Systematic review）最早在 20 世纪初应用于医学研究，但直到 1970 年以后，医学界才普遍认可其优越性和应用性。及至 2000 年前后，这种综述类型的体制逐渐固定下来，子类型也愈加多样。应该说，系统性综述的普及伴随着循证医学的成熟、医学文献的电子化、数据抓取和分析工具的开发等诸多方面的进展。本节将着重介绍系统性综述格式和内容的写作。

2.1 系统性综述的内容要求

系统性综述的研究问题应和临床实践或公共卫生相关，是作者以问题为基础，收集所有已发表或现有的临床研究结果，采用临床流行病学严格评价文献的原则和方法，筛选出符合质量标准的文献，进行定量合成分析，得出综合可靠的结论，以改进临床医疗实践、帮助制订公共卫生政策和指导临床研究方向。如果系统综述包含有 Meta 分析，通常在方法部分，包含有如下小标题：综述框架（Review frame）、研究策略（Study strategy）、研究选择（Study selection）、资格标准（Eligibility criteria）、数据收集（Data collection）、偏倚风险评估（Risk of bias assessment）、Meta 分析（Meta-analysis）和对证据体系的信心（Confidence in the body of evidence）等。

2.2 系统性综述的写作格式

一般来说，系统性综述的文章格式按照摘要（Abstract）、前言（Introduction）、方法（Methods）、结果（Results）、讨论（Discussion）和结论（Conclusion）等部分展开。

2.2.1 摘要

系统性综述的摘要一般要求不超过 200 字，含有目的（Objective）、数据来源（Data sources）、研究选择（Study selection）、数据提取（Data extraction）、数据合成（Data synthesis）和结论（Conclusion/Summary）等副标题，也有的期刊不单独列出副标题，而将副标题里所涉及的内容融合在一起，形成一段完整的摘要。

下面将结合实例来说明摘要里各部分要点的写作。

（1）在"目的"里，需要准确说明综述的主要目标，确定综述是强调病因和诊断、预后、治疗和干预，还是预防，确定综述是高选择性的，即只包括随机对照试验（RCT），还是有更广泛的纳入标准。英文表达常用"aim to …"等描述研究目的。

例 1：This review <u>aims to</u> determine whether depression rates have increased and review evidence for possible explanations.

本综述旨在确定抑郁症发病率是否有所上升，同时回顾文献，寻找可能的解释。

（2）因为系统性综述采纳定量分析的研究方法，所以有的期刊要求在摘要部分重点描述文献数据的收集及处理情况："数据来源"部分主要介绍所使用的数据来源，包括数据选取时间上的限定；"研究选择"部分主要说明所选取的用来具体综述的文献标准，说明所使用的方法，如盲审、共识、多人评审等；"数据提取"部分主要说明如何进行数据提取，包括对质量和有效性的评估。

例 2：We searched the PubMed database for epidemiological studies on ambient temperature and morbidity of noncommunicable diseases published in refereed English journals before 30 June 2020. Forty relevant studies were identified. Of these, 24 examined the relationship between ambient temperature and morbidity, 15 investigated the short-term effects of heat wave on morbidity, and 1 assessed both temperature and heat wave effects.

我们在 PubMed 数据库中搜索了 2020 年 6 月 30 日前在有参考价值的英文期刊上发表的关于环境温度和非传染性疾病发病率的流行病学研究，共有 40 项相关研究。其中，24 项研究了环境温度和发病率之间的关系，15 项研究了热浪对发病率的短期影响，1 项同时评估了温度和热浪的影响。

（3）"数据提取"部分主要介绍了综述的主要结果，并陈述已确定的研究之间差异的主要来源。

例 3：Descriptive and time-series studies were the two main research designs used to investigate the temperature-morbidity relationship. Measurements of temperature exposure and health outcomes were used in these studies differed widely. The majority of studies reported a significant relationship between ambient temperature and total or cause-specific morbidities. However, there were some inconsistencies in the direction and magnitude of nonlinear lag effects. The lag effect of hot temperature on morbidity was shorter (several days) compared with that of cold temperature (up to a few weeks). The temperature-morbidity relationship may be confounded or modified by sociodemographic factors and air pollution.

描述性研究和时间序列研究是用于调查温度与疾病关系的两个主要研究设计。这些研究中使用的温度暴露和健康结果的测量方法差别很大。大多数研究报告称，环境温度与总发病率或特定病因发病率之间存在显著关系。然而，在非线性滞后效应的方向和程度上存在一些不一致。与低温（长达几周）相比，高温对发病率的滞后效应较短（数天）。温度与发病率的关系可能受到社会人口因素和空气污染的影响。

（4）"结论"部分主要陈述最后的结论，以及结论的可推广性和局限性。

例 4：There is a significant short-term effect of ambient temperature on total and cause-specific morbidities. However, further research is needed to determine an appropriate temperature measure, consider a diverse range of morbidities, and to use consistent methodology to make different studies more comparable.

环境温度对总发病率和特定病因发病率有明显的短期影响。不过,需要进一步研究以确定适当的温度测量方法,考虑各种不同的发病率,并使用一致的方法,使不同的研究更具可比性。

2.2.2 前言

系统性综述的前言部分和原创性研究论文类似,但不需要更长的文献调查,只回顾以往的综述文献,并说明本次综述的原因和目的。这里不再赘述。

2.2.3 方法

方法部分可以有和摘要相对应的小标题(如数据来源、研究选择、数据提取等),并应包括明确的纳入和排除标准,以及作为数据来源的数据库和其他正式登记簿、会议记录、参考文献列表和试验作者的具体说明。这里应提供完整的检索策略,以便于后面的研究者效仿。如果认为篇幅过长,无法在文章中发表,可以选择以电子文档的形式在附录中出现。

例 5:We estimated deaths and disability-adjusted life years attributable to the independent effects of 67 risk factors and clusters of risk factors for 21 regions in 2010 and 2020. We estimated exposure distributions for each year, region, sex, and age group, and relative risks per unit of exposure by systematically reviewing and synthesizing published and unpublished data. We used these estimates, together with estimates of cause-specific deaths and DALYs from the Global Burden of Disease Study 2020, to calculate the burden attributable to each risk factor exposure compared with the theoretical-minimum-risk exposure. We incorporated uncertainty in disease burden, relative risks, and exposures into our estimates of attributable burden.

我们估算了 2010 年和 2020 年 21 个地区图 67 种风险因素和风险因素群的独立影响而导致的死亡人数和伤残调整生命年数。我们通过系统回顾和综合已发表及未发表的数据,估算了各年份、地区、性别和年龄组的暴露分布,以及每单位暴露的相对风险。我们利用这些估算值以及《2020 年全球疾病负担研究》对特定病因死亡人数和伤残调整生命年数(DALYs)的估算值,计算出与理论最低风险暴露值相比,每个风险因素暴露造成的负担。我们将疾病负担、相对风险和暴露的不确定性纳入了可归因负担的估算中。

系统性综述的结果(Results)、讨论(Discussion)和结论(Conclusion)的写作方法可参照原创文章相应部分的写作,此处将不赘述。

各类期刊对系统综述的格式要求并不完全一样,文献综述类文章的特点决定了文章里存在着大量的对前人研究成果的引述和评价。如何评述这些研究成果并表达作者自己的观点也是综述类文章需要注意的问题。

第三节 医学文献综述的语言特征

3.1 医学文献综述标题的语言特征

与一般论文的标题相比,医学文献综述的标题表述往往比较概念化,经常运用"研究进展""研究现状""新概念""重新评估"等短语,有的在主标题或副标题中直接注明"Review of ..."或"A review of ...",有时 review 前面还会加上限定语,从最常使用的 systematic,到 comprehensive、scoping、rapid 等。其次,由于综述性文献与 Meta 分析研究之间有着千丝万缕的联系,Meta-analysis 等词在综述标题中也不鲜见,使读者一眼就能看出这篇文献的类型。同时,综述标题应包括当前主题的关键词或其衍生词,以提高文章的检出率。

例 1:A systematic review on the role of eicosanoid pathways in rheumatoid arthritis

类风湿性关节炎中类二十烷途径作用的系统综述

例 2:Association of brain-derived neurotrophic factor gene polymorphisms with body mass index:A systematic review and Meta-analysis

脑源性神经营养因子基因多态性与体重指数的相关性:系统综述和荟萃分析

此外,综述的基本目的之一是温故而知新,因此在回顾研究历史的基础上往往会更进一步介绍学科的最新进展,因此标题中会有诸如"update""new""emerging"等词。

例 3:Emerging concepts in liquid biopsies

液体活检中的新概念

例 4:Impact of comorbidities on gout and hyperuricaemia:an update on prevalence and treatment options

并发症对痛风和高尿酸血症的影响:发病率和治疗方案的最新进展

3.2 医学文献综述摘要的语言特征

医学文献综述的摘要多是指示性摘要(Indicative abstract),一般只指出研究要点,引导读者阅读全文。有的评论性综述没有摘要部分。但国内文献综述,大多包括摘要和关键词。文献综述摘要部分的时态有一般现在时、一般过去时和现在完成时等。

例 5:Knee arthroplasty is commonly performed in the case of advanced osteoarthritis, and deep joint infections represent a severe complication following surgery. A 4-year retrospective cohort study was conducted to determine the incidence and risk factors for such surgical site infections. Of the 2439 patients <u>included</u> in the study, 84 of them (3.4%) developed infections. Postoperative bleeding, Ahlback's disease, obesity, smoking, and male gender <u>were</u> independent risk factors that should be considered when caring for those patients.

【分析】

（1）这段摘要的第一句话用 ... is commonly performed in the case of ... 和 ... represent ... 描述了深部关节感染（deep joint infections），时态为一般现在时。（2）第二句话交代了为期四年的研究重点，即手术部位感染的发病率和危险因素。时态为一般过去时，动词是 was 和 developed。（3）第三句是研究结果，时态为一般过去时，其中 included 是过去分词，意指"被纳入研究的"。（4）第四句提到了护理这些病人时，应该考虑（... should be considered ... ）的一些独立危险因素，两句都是一般过去时。

【实用表达】

- advanced osteoarthritis 晚期骨关节炎
- joint infections 关节感染
- complication following surgery 术后的并发症
- retrospective cohort study 回顾性队列研究
- incidence and risk factors 发病率和危险因素
- postoperative bleeding 术后出血
- independent risk factor 独立风险因素

【参考译文】

膝关节置换术是晚期骨关节炎患者的常见手术，深部关节感染是手术后的严重并发症。一项为期 4 年的回顾性队列研究旨在确定此类手术部位感染的发生率和风险因素。在纳入研究的 2 439 名患者中，有 84 人（3.4%）发生了深部感染。术后出血、阿尔贝克氏病、肥胖、吸烟和男性，是护理这些患者时应考虑的独立风险因素。

例 6：More profound understanding of the relationship between the burnout and the limbic system function can provide better insight into brain structures associated with the burnout syndrome. The objective of this review is to explore all evidence of limbic brain structures associated with the burnout syndrome. In total, 13 studies were selected. Four of them applied the neuroimaging technology to investigate the sizes/volumes of the limbic brain structures of burnout patients. Six other studies were to investigate the hypothalamus-pituitary-adrenal (HPA) axis of burnout patients. Based on the results of the studies on the HPA-axis and neuroimaging of the limbic brain structures, one can see great impact of the chronic occupational stress on the limbic structures in terms of HPA dysregulation, a decrease of BDNF, impaired neurogenesis and limbic structures atrophy. It can be concluded that chronic stress inhibits the feedback control pathway in the HPA axis, causes the decrease of brain-derived neurotrophic factor（BDNF），then impaired neurogenesis and eventually neuron atrophy.

【分析】

本摘要第一句用... understanding of ... can provide better insight into ... 描述了综述的意义，即"对倦怠和边缘系统功能之间关系的更为深刻的理解，有助于人们更好地洞察与倦怠综合征相关的大脑结构"。第二句用 The objective of this review is to ... 描述了综述的目的，即"探索与倦怠综合征相关的边缘脑结构的所有证据"。接下来的第三、四句描述了综述的过程和手段，动词的时态为一般过去时。第五句廓清了现有研究的成果，作者用 one can see ... 提示读者注意本课题找到的依据。最后一句用了被动语态 It can be concluded that ... 描述了结论，that 后面句子的谓语动词用的是一般现在时 inhibits、causes，表示结论具有普遍意义。

【实用表达】

- profound understanding 深刻理解
- limbic system function 边缘系统功能
- the burnout syndrome 倦怠综合征
- neuroimaging technology 神经成像技术
- chronic occupational stress 慢性职业压力
- limbic structures atrophy 边缘结构萎缩
- neuron atrophy 神经元萎缩

【参考译文】

更为深刻地理解倦怠和边缘系统功能之间的关系，有助于人们更好地洞察与倦怠综合征相关的大脑结构。这篇综述的目的是探索与倦怠综合征相关的边缘脑结构的所有证据。总共选择了13项研究。其中四项应用神经成像技术研究了倦怠患者边缘脑结构的大小/体积。另外六项研究是调查倦怠患者的下丘脑-垂体-肾上腺轴。根据边缘脑结构的羟丙基肾上腺轴和神经影像的研究结果，可以看到慢性职业压力对边缘结构的巨大影响，表现为羟丙基肾上腺失调、BDNF下降、神经发生受损和边缘结构萎缩。可以得出结论，慢性应激抑制 HPA 轴中的反馈控制途径，导致脑源性神经营养因子（BDNF）减少，然后损害神经发生并最终导致神经元萎缩。

3.3 医学文献综述前言的语言特征

文献综述的前言主要包括两部分：提出问题、说明综述要讨论的范围和内容。前言不宜太长，一般为100—200词。前言部分应该廓清当前综述的价值，如有必要还可阐明与他人的综述有何区别。

*例 7：*Today blood biochemical laboratory tests are essential elements to the diagnosis and monitoring of the treatment of diseases. However, many researchers have suggested saliva as an preferable diagnostic material. The collection of saliva is simple, painless, cheap and safe, both for patients and medical staff. An additional advantage of saliva is the fact that it may be retrieved several times a day, which makes repeat analysis much easier. Furthermore, saliva has very high durability. Although 94%–99% of salivary content is water, saliva also contains numerous cellular elements and many organic and inorganic substances, including most biological markers present in the blood and urine that may be used in the early detection and monitoring of many dental and general diseases.

【分析】

这部分介绍了研究的背景,第一句用… are essential elements to … 引出研究的主题。第二句用 However 指出之前研究者对于唾液作为更好的诊断材料的观点,谓语动词用了现在完成时 have suggested。第三、四句的谓语动词时态大多为一般现在时,简要展示了唾液作为诊断材料的优越性,属于客观事实的陈述;其中被动语态(may be retrieved)和非限定性定语从句(which makes …),凸显了学术英语的语言特点。第五句用 furthermore 表示递进,进一步凸显唾液样本的稳定性能。最后一句说明唾液对于一般疾病的早期检测和监测的意义,其中被动语态… may be used … 陈述了客观事实。

【实用表达】

- blood biochemical laboratory tests 血液生化实验室检测
- diagnosis and monitoring of the treatment of diseases 诊断和监测疾病治疗
- patients and medical staff 病人和医护人员
- additional advantage 另一个优点
- cellular elements 细胞元素
- organic and inorganic substances 有机和无机物
- biological markers 生物标记
- blood and urine 血液和尿液
- early detection and monitoring 早期检测和监测
- general diseases 一般疾病

【参考译文】

如今,血液生化实验室检测是诊断和监测疾病治疗的基本要素。然而,许多研究人员认为唾液是更好的诊断材料。对病人和医护人员来说,采集唾液简单、无痛、便宜且安全。唾液的另一个优点是每天可以多次采集,这使得重复分析更加容易。此外,唾液具有很高的持久性。虽然唾液的 94%—99% 是水,但唾液也含有大量的细胞元素和许多有机和无机物,包括血液和尿液中存在的大多数生物标记,这些标记可用于许多牙科疾病和一般疾病的早期检测和监测。

3.4　医学文献综述中述评的语言特征

述评部分是文献综述的主体,是作者对众多文献资料进行系统分析、提炼精华到形成自己观点的关键部分,一般可根据分析的步骤加小标题辅助说明。综述是"对研究的再研究",虽然传统的叙述性评论倚重于理论思辨,但也需呈现清晰的研究方法。系统性综述则会描述检索的关键词、筛选的数据库以及为文献检索选择的时间范围,还应解释研究的纳入和排除标准等。动词时态常用一般现在时或现在完成时,而回顾性述评常用一般过去时或过去完成时。下面是某篇综述述评部分的节选:

例 8:

Literature review on Legionella

A standard literature review starts by searching online subscription-based websites that provide scientific citation indexing services. However, guidelines, standards, and regulations cannot be found in this way. For this article, a literature search was performed only with the aim to identify the most influential Legionella researchers.

In Figure 2, research published over the years about Legionella is shown. When performing a literature search for the key word "Legionella" in scientific journals in all fields—meaning the word "Legionella" appears at least once in the whole article—15,589 results were found. Research on Legionella has been published since the 1970s. The number of articles has been increasing since 1979. When looking for the more specific key word "Legionella pneumophila" (all combinations of capitals) in all fields, 7,615 results were found. The curve is an offset of the curve in Figure 2, meaning publications follow a similar evolution over time.

Comparison with other references

Many of the published guidelines and standards are not necessarily evidence-based. That is why, for each common item that has been identified, references to scientific (clinical) studies that support the importance of these items are given, if available. The precision, accuracy, and effectiveness of ways to estimate the risk of higher Legionella numbers have only rarely been empirically assessed in practice, although there is a broad consensus regarding the impact of these risk factors.

Discussion

Comparing frameworks can be a first step on the path to future unification of Legionella regulations. Current regulations involve a wide range of climatologic circumstances. Still, the same measures are recommended in different environmental circumstances worldwide because it is the characteristics of the DHW system that dominate over different climatic conditions. Clearer and more uniform and unambiguous regulations will facilitate their implementation. Finally, we can ask the question, "Do we have clear, uniform, and unambiguous Legionella guidelines and regulations?" The answer is obviously that we do not. However, despite different regulatory frameworks, there is a broad unification of principles.

【分析】

所选例文第一部分第一段的头两句描述的是当前文献综述的现状,用的是一般现在时 starts、cannot be found,第三句在提到当前文献的搜索方法时,用的一般过去时 was performed。第二段的第一句在提到文章中的图表时,用了一般现在时 is,这个原则在前几章介绍学术论文的撰写时已经提到,不再赘述。接下来的几句话分别包含一般现在时、一般过去时、现在完成时和现在完成进行时,用来描述按本研究的方法输入关键词"军团菌"后,出现的检索结果。同时,也出现了学术英语论文里常见的被动语态,如:were found、has been published 等。

第二部分是对比其他参考文献存在的方法上的缺点,提出本研究对于军团菌的综述的意义所在,用的是一般现在时和现在完成时。

在第三部分讨论里,提出要有更清晰、更统一、更明确的框架来实施军团菌法规。时态为一般现在时和将来时,如... can be a first step、... are recommended、... will facilitate ... 等。同时值得注意的是,这部分语义的逻辑连接手段,如 can be、still、because、finally、however 等,使得综述的语言表达显得客观、严谨。

【实用表达】

- online subscription-based websites 在线订阅网站
- scientific citation indexing services 科学引文索引服务
- guidelines, standards, and regulations 指导方针、标准和条例
- literature search 文献检索
- scientific journals 科学期刊
- in all fields 所有领域
- an offset of the curve 曲线的偏移
- follow a similar evolution 遵循类似的演变
- evidence-based 基于证据的,循证的
- precision, accuracy, and effectiveness 精确性、准确性和有效性
- empirically assessed in practice 在应用中实证
- a broad consensus 广泛的共识
- frameworks 框架
- a wide range of 广泛的
- dominate over 主宰着
- climatic conditions 气候条件
- uniform and unambiguous regulations 统一、明确的法规

- regulatory frameworks 监管框架
- a broad unification of principles 广泛统一的原则

3.5 医学文献综述结论的语言特征

结论部分要提供对结果的解释并提出专家意见，从而引导读者把握当前证据。如果确实没有足够的证据来得出客观的结论，则需说明，可讨论纳入文献的局限性、偏差以及综述过程本身的局限性。综述的结论部分对领域内其他学者的未来研究、临床实践，乃至公共政策制定有着重大的导向意义。

例 9：Hospitals worldwide are concerned about infection control and have implemented numerous patient safety protocols to combat horizontal transmission of infectious agents. The findings of this review suggest that provider attire is a potential source of transmission for pathogenic bacteria in health care settings. However, data confirming a direct link between provider attire and HAIs remains limited. It seems appropriate to develop protocols needed to reduce contamination of both white coats and surgical scrubs. The suggestions outlined in this article, based on available evidence, may serve as a guideline for health care professionals and hospital systems to reduce the spread of bacterial pathogens, including MDROs, that have the potential to precipitate hospital-acquired infections.

【分析】

结论是对整篇综述的总结，通常会在第一句里重申一下研究的关键词，如本文里的 infection control、horizontal transmission、infectious agents。同时会用 The findings of this review suggest that ... 的句式来阐述综述的结论。接着用 However, ... remains limited 的句式来说明本研究存在的问题，用 It seems appropriate to ... 的句式，对未来的研究提出建议。最后用 The suggestions outlined in this article may serve as a guideline for ... 肯定了本综述的意义所在。

【实用短语】

- patient safety protocols 患者安全协议
- horizontal transmission 横向传播
- infectious agents 传染媒介
- health care settings 卫生保健环境
- health care professionals 卫生保健专业人员
- hospital systems 医院系统
- bacterial pathogens 细菌病原体

【参考译文】

世界各地的医院都很关注感染控制，并实施了许多患者安全协议，以防止传染媒介的横向传播。综述的结果表明,医护人员的着装是卫生保健环境中致病菌潜在传播源。然而,确认医疗人员服装和 HAIs 之间有直接联系的数据仍然有限。现今,制定减少白大褂和手术服污染所需的规程似乎是合适的。本文中概述的建议,基于现有的证据,可以作为卫生保健专业人员和医院系统的指导方针,以减少细菌病原体的传播,包括有可能加剧院内获得性感染的多药耐药菌。

第四节　医学文献综述常用句型

本节就叙述性综述和系统性综述的共性,结合实例就如何"综",如何"述"的问题,即如何引用、叙述及评价前人的研究成果、研究的不足,引出新的科研问题,对进一步的研究工作进行展望等常见句型结合范例进行解释。

4.1　如何"综"?

（1）在叙述前人的研究时,可采用直接引用的方式。

例 1：According to Nissan H（2021）,"The broader effects of climate change on local livelihoods, food security, and migration may increase population vulnerability to the disease."

Nissan（2021）认为,"气候变化对当地生计、食品安全以及移民的更广泛影响,可能会增加人口对疾病的易感性"。

例 2：As Villalobos Prats E（2020）has indicated："To help address the additional burden of health care delivery created by a changing climate, health professionals can advocate for more climate-resilient health systems."

正如 Prats E Villalobos（2020）所指出的,"为帮助解决气候变化给医疗保健服务带来的额外负担,医疗卫生专业人员可以倡导建立更具气候适应能力的医疗卫生系统"。

需要注意的是直接引用的句子在文献综述文章里所占比例有限,所以要事先查看所要发表文章的期刊要求,以确定直接引用的句子数量和比例。

（2）在叙述前人的研究时,可采取总结性叙述或概括性叙述,即间接引用的方法,或在句末尾加注符号,在文章后的参考文献中表明具体出处。

例 3：According to Nissan H（2021）, the broader effects of climate change on local livelihoods, food security, and migration may increase population vulnerability to the disease.

这个例子是例 1 采用间接引用后的另外一种引述方法。

例 4：Carpenter and Gardner showed a relationship between sulphury deposition levels and SIDS in England and Wales.

Carpenter 和 Gardner 的研究表明,英格兰和威尔士的硫化物沉积水平和 SIDS 之间存在关系。

与例 4 画线的单词有类似功能的还有 studied、investigated、claimed、mentioned、stated 等词。

例 5：<u>Cama's 2021 paper on</u> factors associated with severe disease in children <u>proposed</u> that high temperatures increase the number of admissions for bacterial diarrheal disease.

Cama 在 2021 年关于儿童严重疾病相关因素的论文中提出,高温会增加细菌性腹泻疾病的入院人数。

（3）在叙述前人的研究时,只提及研究内容,在句末括号里标注出处。

例 6：Patients with chronic hand eczema, vitiligo, or atopic eczema presented more anxiety than healthy controls (Kouris et al. ,2015；Hamidizadeh et al. , 2020；Treudler et al. , 2020).

与健康对照组相比,慢性手部湿疹、白癜风或特应性湿疹患者表现出更多的焦虑 (Kouris et al. , 2015；Hamidizadeh et al. , 2020；Treudler et al. , 2020)。

例 7：About 30% of cystic fibrosis patients (Havermans et al. , 2008；Olveira et al. , 2016) presented severe anxious symptoms and 15% of those with neurofibromatosis type 1 described moderate-severe anxiety (Doser et al. , 2020).

约 30%的囊性纤维化患者出现了严重的焦虑症状 (Havermans et al. , 2008；Olveira et al. , 2016),15%的神经纤维瘤病 1 型患者出现了中度—重度焦虑症状 (Doser et al. , 2020)。

（4）直接提及研究结果,依照其在文中出现的先后顺序,在引用处右上角用数字标出,同时按引用先后顺序将参考文献排列于文末。

例 8：Evidence suggests that allergic respiratory diseases such as bronchial asthma have become more common worldwide in recent years[4]；

有证据表明,近年来支气管哮喘等过敏性呼吸道疾病在全球范围内越来越常见。[4]

References

4. United Nations Environment Programme and WHO Report. Air pollution in the world's megacities. A report from the U. N. environment programme and WHO. Environment 1994；36：5 - 37.

例 9：A study in the Netherlands[17], showed that atopic children with bronchial hyper-responsiveness (BHR) are at risk of increased respiratory symptoms during episodes of air pollution.

References

17. Boezen HM，van der Zee SC，Postma DS et al. Effects of ambient air pollution on upper and lower respiratory symptoms and peak expiratory flow in children. Lancet 1999；353：874 - 878.

荷兰的一项研究[17]显示,患有支气管高反应性(BHR)的特应性儿童在空气污染期间有增加呼吸道症状的风险。

4.2 如何"述"?

综述是就特定主题的研究进行回顾,描述共识领域、查明当前证据状况、提示进一步研究的方向。综述类文章的起点是明确研究的问题,然后依靠文献的获取和综合,获得可信的数据和资料,是为"综",接着进入"述"的环节。"述"需要对所综述的内容进行综合、分析、评价,将归纳、整理的科学事实和资料进行排列和必要的分析,对有争论的问题介绍各家观点或学说,进行比较,指出问题的焦点和可能的发展趋势,并提出自己的看法。综述应有作者的观点,否则就不成为综述,只是文献记录了。

下面将结合实例介绍评、述的常用句型:

例 10：Previous literature <u>has illustrated that</u> U-、V-、or J-shaped patterns change with the minimum morbidity or mortality at a certain temperature or temperature range，with increased morbidity or mortality below and above the threshold.

以前的文献说明,在某一温度或温度范围内,U 型、V 型或 J 型的发病率或死亡率最低,低于或高于阈值时,发病率或死亡率增加。

Previous literature has illustrated that ... 是将"综"和"述"结合在一起对既往文献评述的常用句型,这里常用的动词除了 illustrate,还有 demonstrate、prove、propose、consider 等。

例 11：The association between maternal smoking and SIDS <u>has been well established</u>, and current knowledge also suggests that smoking contributes significantly to indoor-air pollution.

母亲吸烟与婴儿猝死综合征之间的关系已经得到证实,目前的知识还表明,吸烟也是造成室内空气污染的重要原因。

例 12：<u>The existing studies to date have made an important contribution to</u> the field by providing intriguing，preliminary evidence for the role of sleep as a mediator.

到目前为止,现有的研究为睡眠作为媒介的作用提供了有趣的初步证据,对该领域做出了重要贡献。

句中下画线部分的句式是对当前某领域研究的一个积极的评价。

例 13：<u>No</u> longitudinal studies <u>have been conducted to</u> date to assess the effect of air pollution on SIDS.

迄今为止，尚未开展纵向研究来评估空气污染对婴儿猝死综合征的影响。

本例用 No ... have been conducted to ... 的句式指出既往文献的研究空白。

例 14：The effects of intrauterine exposures to episodes of elevated pollution and/or prolonged exposures to modest levels <u>need further examination as no study has examined</u> the relative importance of pre- and post-natal exposures to air pollution on the occurrence of SIDS.

宫内暴露于高污染的事件和/或长期暴露于适度的污染水平的影响需要进一步研究，因为还没有研究探讨产前和产后暴露于空气污染对发生婴儿猝死综合征的相对重要性。

本例中用 ... need further examination as no study has examined ... 的句式提出了未来研究的方向及原因所在。

例 15：This article <u>would have been more</u> convincing if the author had related his findings to previous work on the topic.

如果作者能将他的研究结果与之前有关该主题的工作联系起来，这篇文章会更有说服力。

本句用 ... would have been more ... 的结构委婉地指出所综述的文献在方法或内容上需要改进的地方。

第五节　练习巩固

1. 阅读下列医学综述节选，选文中出现了 5 处时态错误，请找出并改正。

Gaucher disease（GD，OMIM 230800）is a rare hereditary autosomal recessive disorder characterized by a multisystemic condition resulting from mutations in the gene encoding glucocerebrosidase（acid β-glucosidase）. GD is the most common of the lysosomal storage diseases. A decreased glucocerebrosidase activity leads to accumulation of glucocerebroside（glucosylceramide）in the lysosomes of macrophages, inducing Gaucher cell infiltration of the bone marrow and visceral organs. As a consequence, a complex disorder is produced with hepatosplenomegaly, anemia and thrombocytopenia, bone involvement and less commonly, lung or CNS involvement. In addition, pro-inflammatory cytokines and the adaptive immune system appear to be involved and hyperferritinemia, hypergammaglobulinemia, altered calcium homeostasis and metabolic syndrome are frequently associated with GD.

Ferritin is an iron-binding protein that stores iron in a biologically available form for vital cellular processes and protects proteins, lipids and DNA from the potential toxicity of iron. Ferritin plays a role in a large number of conditions including inflammatory, neurodegenerative and malignant diseases. In GD there has been an increased amount of iron in Gaucher cells, with no evidence of increased avidity between iron and glucocerebroside storage material. The excess of iron induced a conversion of hydrogen peroxide free radical that is very toxic to tissues through oxidation of proteins, peroxidation of membrane lipids and modification of nucleic acids. There are several clinical situations in which there is an excess of iron in tissue stores such as in thalassemia, myelodysplastic syndromes or in patients who will receive hematopoietic stem cell transplantation, and require repeated transfusions. The chronic diseases in which the mononuclear macrophage system is committed, as in some storage diseases such as GD have hyperferritinemia. In these situations, the possible damage to the heart and liver introduce a negative factor to therapy outcomes.

Iron regulation was subject to the blocking of intestinal absorption effectors by hepcidin, a circulating peptide produced by hepatocytes that is influenced by inflammatory cytokines. Circulating hepcidin has exerted its effect by binding to membrane ferroportin, a cellular iron exporter. In iron overload conditions, the increase of hepcidin levels inhibits intestinal iron absorption, whereas the peptide appears diminished in the absence of iron stores. Hepcidin is upregulated by multiple factors, several of which are involved in GD such as cytokines, which are known to increase transcription of the hepcidin gene and are elevated in patients with GD. It is speculated that disruption of iron control mechanisms contributes to the development of some pathologic conditions such as inflammation, neurodegeneration, metabolic disorders and cancer, all of which occur frequently in GD.

Challenges remain to studying modifications induced in the biomarkers, hepcidin level and iron profile of GD patients under therapy. These changes after chelator therapy in patients with hyperferritinemia and liver iron overload could prevent other inflammatory dysfunctions.

2. 阅读下列医学综述节选，用所给关联词，使句子语意连贯、语篇完整。

| thereafter | however | as well as | also | on the other hand |

Clinical manifestations of FXIIID encompass a wide-variety of bleeding symptoms. These can be either spontaneous or provoked bleeds after trauma, surgery, dental operation, etc. In line with appropriate diagnostic laboratory tests, clinical and familial history can be used to assist the diagnostic process. In the present study, characterizing UCB, along with a variety of other features were observed in neonates who were diagnosed with FXIII-A deficiency. ICH was observed in 48.1% of the patients, while familial history was positive in 66.6%. Emphases on timely diagnosis in suspected cases are essential to reduce morbidity and mortality. (1) _____, type of delivery may trigger bleeding symptoms such as CNS bleeding in the affected patients. CS might be superior to NVD, if fetus is affected with FXIIID, but the mother's coagulation status has to be taken into consideration. In this study, there was no statistically significant difference between the type of delivery and CNS bleeding which might be due to low number of included subjects. (2) _____, manipulated or complicated NVD using forceps or vacuum would be associated with higher risk of CNS bleeding compared to CS in rare coagulation disorders.

Despite being the country with the most prevalence of FXIIID around the world, studies on neonates with FXIIID and their clinical presentations are scare in Iran. The most common clinical feature amongst Iranian patients with FXIIID is UCB followed by ICH, and hematoma, which was reported amongst neonates in the present study. However, bleedings that has the highest impact on the lives of patients, are CNS bleeding that incur a high rate of mortality and morbidity. Nearly 30% of patients suffering from FXIIID may experience hemorrhaging episodes in the brain that can be encountered at any stage of life in the affected patients. Our study can be a guide for physicians and neonatal nursing care. Detecting positive family history led us to be highly suspicious and consider prenatal diagnosis (PND), if accessible. Positive PND renders preferred CS over NVD, which prevents further complications. In this study, all the patients were treated with factor XIII concentrates on the first presentation and it was repeated two days later, and (3) _____, prophylactic therapy was initiated at a low dose of 10 IU/kg every 4 weeks, leading to an acceptable result.

As we performed in our patients, continuous factor replacement therapy is the primary therapeutic approach in patients with severe factor XIIID. The relatively long half-life of administrated FXIII concentrates (7 – 14 days) allows prophylactic factor replacement strategy to be successfully implemented in deficient patients. However, the life-span of infused FXIII is also dependent on both dose and frequency of administrated concentration. In this study, after initial clinical evaluation, we performed general first-line coagulation tests followed by a molecular diagnostic assay. The first line coagulation tests including: PT, APTT, BT, fibrinogen assay, and platelet count were within normal rage in these patients. However, definite diagnosis, using specific factor assay, functional or antigenic level assessment, (4) _____, clot solubility test, are required since negative molecular screening test cannot rule out FXIIID. （5）_____, clot solubility test is no longer recommended due to lack of specificity. More than 150 mutations reported to be responsible for FXIIID worldwide. Amongst these, Trp187Arg (exon 4, C. 559T> C) mutation is the most common, and the only reported mutation in southeastern Iran. In Iran, molecular diagnostic approach for detecting RBDs is not routine due to limited resources. This approach is mainly confined to prenatal diagnosis centers, especially our center, which provides screening programs for parents.

3. 按照括号里的中文提示，完成句子，注意正确运用时态和语态。

（1）This review _____（评估了）the evidence of a link between exposure to ambient air pollution and the incidence of SIDS.

（2）In the past few years, much a etiological and pathogenic research _____ _____（被研究过了）in the attempt to determine the relationship between the effects of air pollution and human health.

（3）These studies _____（确认了）the general risks of temperature as well as temperature extremes in multiple areas over time, using different research designs.

（4）Other outbreaks of asthma caused by soybean dust pollution _____（记载于）the Spanish cities of Tarragona and Cartagena.

（5）Many of these reviews specifically _____（关注）the sleep characteristics of individuals with posttraumatic stress disorder (PTSD) or acute stress disorder.

（6）Current literature _____（阐释了）that malaria among children is also affected by temperature extremes.

（7）This review has several _____（意义）for clinical practice and public policy.

（8）This study is considered one of the largest asthma studies _____（做过的）involving adults, adolescents, and children as young as 4 years old.

（9）Deteriorating health of modern populations via the obesity epidemic is a likely _____（影响因素）to a rising prevalence of depression.

（10）The management of gallstone ileus is _____（有争议的）.

（11）_____（基于本综述里所收集的数据）and general research on how exposure to violence influences child health and development, a conceptual model is proposed.

（12）A recent study by Koren, Arnon, Lavie, and Klein (2002) assessed sleep more thoroughly using the Mini Sleep Questionnaire (Zomer, Peled, Rubin, & Lavie, 1987) and found sleep disturbance to _____ _____（有很强的预后意义）.

（13）Several studies have _____（系统地研究了）the content of

the nightmares experienced by people with PTSD.

(14) Large scale study analyzing children by cause-specific outcomes in temperature extremes _____（将会有益处）for making future adaptation strategies.

(15) Ball et al. used the same approach of Molfino _____
_____（回避了早期研究的局限性）.

(16) In contrast to the significant increase in the number of recent studies testing father effects models，_____
_____（仅仅有少数研究已经测试了儿童影响模式）.

(17) _____
（一项前瞻性研究的系统性回顾）found a reciprocal cause-and-effect relationship between obesity/overweight and depression.

(18) There has been much progress，but countless questions circling depression and its origins _____（仍然没有得到解答）.

(19) The role in influencing risk of chronic diseases and depression _____
_____（值得研究）.

(20) _____（有大量的证据支持）
the influence of individual nutrients on mental health.

医学英语应用文写作

第一章　个人简历

第一节　简历的分类和内容

　　从医学生的角度来看,个人简历大致分为两种:一种是因继续学习深造而需要到国外读研读博的留学简历,一种是求职简历。两者因为目的不同,侧重点会有所不同。留学简历中最重要的内容是教育背景,而求职简历最突出的应该是工作经历。除此之外,英语考试成绩在留学简历中占据重要位置,是必须呈现出来的。而求职简历则视申请的工作单位要求,选择要不要填上英语成绩。因此,在内容上,两种简历基本相似,只是部分的侧重点有所变化。

　　留学简历和求职简历一般包含个人信息、申请的职位或目标、工作经历、教育背景、发表的论文、英语考试成绩、获得的各种奖励和荣誉、业余活动/个人技能等基本内容。其中,业余活动/个人技能、发表的论文为简历的非必要内容,可视具体情况进行取舍。如上所述,英语考试成绩在求职简历中也非必要内容。

　　特别注意的是,简历中的时间顺序应该是倒叙,接近现在的事情写在前面,之前的事情写在后面。

- 个人信息(Personal information)
- 申请的职位或目标(Objective)
- 工作经历/科研经历(Working experience/Research experience)
- 教育背景(Education)
- 语言掌握情况(Language proficiency)
- 获得的各种奖励和荣誉(Honors & Awards)
- 业余活动/个人技能(Activities/Skills)

第二节　简历的语法结构

　　个人简历主要是让录取学校或者用人单位快速而又全方位地了解学生,因此,通常使用各种形式的短语,避免复杂的句子。从语法结构上说,个人简历比较青睐平行结构。平行结构是表达复杂概念的一种有效方法,能使复杂的文本更易于阅读、理解和记忆。工整的结构,能使语言表达简洁明晰,并突出重点内容。

2.1 名词短语平行

例1:

AWARDS & HONORS

2008—2012	Outstanding Student Scholarship
2008	First prize, Anhui Medical Skills Contest
2007	Second prize, National Medical Skills Contest

WORKING EXPERIENCE

2020—2022	Interpreter and guide for foreign visiting scholars
2017—2020	Teaching assistant in biology laboratory
	President of the Student Union

SKILLS

Fluent English

Proficient computer skills

Great ability in intercommunication

2.2 形容词短语平行

例2:

Language Proficiency and Computer Application Skills

Able to speak and write fluently in Chinese and English

Proficient in Microsoft Windows, Word, Excel, and Power Point

Computer Skills

Skilled in using various types of web-designing software

Well-versed in Microsoft 2000

Proficient in C, C++, and Java

2.3 -ed 短语平行

例3:

RESEARCH EXPERIENCE:

2010—Present   Biology Engineering Designer, Nanjing Medical University
Participated in the "Optimal Control System" as part of a national level project sponsored by National Natural Fund
Programmed a three-level BP neural network with Visual C++

Simulated the process with software

EDUCATION：

Sept. 18—July. 22   Bachelor of Medicine，Shanghai Medical University

Majored in Clinical Medicine

Minored in Psychiatry

EXPERIENCE：

September 2020—Present

Team Member

Conducted extensive research on Depression in Young People

March 1997—July 2020

Research Assistant

Conducted research on Acute Respiratory Distress Syndrome in Young People

2.4 -ing 短语平行

例 4：

EXPERIENCE：

2017—2020 American Medical Equipment Company（Shanghai）

Sales Executive

Selling medical equipment in Shanghai and Hangzhou

Providing after-sales services

2020—present   Institute of Medicine，Chinese Academy of Sciences（Beijing）

Team Member

Conducting medical experiments

Writing and publishing research findings

例 5：

Honors and Activities：

2020—Present   Organizing volunteering activity in the Fourth Hospital in Hefei

2017   Receiving Outstanding Student Scholarship

第三节 举例说明

例 1：留学申请简历

Ms. ZHAO，Lili

Address：Room 202，Building 3，Anhui Medical University，Shushan District，

Hefei，China

    Tel：0086-0051-636xxxxx

    Mobile：0086-138xxxxxxx

    E-mail：Zhaolili@ yahoo. com

    Objective：

To enter a Master program in Pharmacy of California University

    Education：

Sept. 2018—Present   Bachelor degree in Anhui Medical University

Major：Pharmacy

Overall GPA：3. 8/4. 0

    Honors&Awards：

2023	First Prize in English Speaking Contest in Anhui Medical University
2021—2022	First Class Scholarship
2021	Third-place in Innovation and Entrepreneurship Competition in Anhui Province

    Experience：

2022—2023	Mengniu Dairy Co. Ltd（Hefei） Research assistant Participated in the market research project Designed questionnaire and sample surveys
2020—2021	Taught in the school of Mentally Retarded Children in Hefei
2019	Volunteered at the Elderly Welfare House in Hefei

    Standardized Tests：

| Aug. 2022 | TOEFL：637 |
| Apr. 2021 | GRE：2140 |

例2：求职简历

Mr. ZHOU，Deng

Address：Room 504，Building 15，Huyue Community，Feili District，Hainan，China

Mobile：0086-180xxxxxxx

E-mail：Hope2010@ yahoo. com

    Objective：

To work as a dentist in Renmin Hospital and utilize professional skills to improve client satisfaction

    Education：

Sept. 2008—July 2011   Master degree in Nanjing Medical University

Sept. 2003—July 2008   Bachelor degree in Anhui Medical University

Overall GPA：3. 8/4. 0

Experience：

2021—Present	Xinhua Dental Solution Hospital—Dentist
Responsibilities：	Examining X-rays
	Filling teeth cavities
	Straightening teeth
	Educating patients on how to prevent teeth-related diseases
2011—2021	Feixi Clinic—Intern Dentist
Responsibilities：	Providing preventive and suitable treatments for mouth and teeth problems
	Providing dental care to the patients

第四节　练习巩固

1. 请将下列简历中的句子利用平行结构通顺简洁化，必要时可进行信息筛选。

（1）Education：

×× University，Sept. 2000—June 2005

Major in Clinical Medicine

Major GPA：3. 8/4. 0

Honors：

Got Outstanding Student Scholarship from 2000—2003

Associate Chairman of Student Union for my department

As Class representative，I am responsible for organizing class activities

（2）Experience：

Sept. 2007—Oct. 2009：Sydney Senior High School，Australia

I was chosen from 500 students to study in this overseas school as an exchange student. During this period，I learnt a lot from my foreign classmates.

Obtained more knowledge about Australia.

My spoken English was much better when I came back from Australia.

（3）Working Experience

Sept. 2000，interpreter in China International Trade Fair for Sanitation and Heating

Teaching Assistant of two students in the high school in 2001

Research Assistant in Lab. of Biology in 2002

2. 根据自己的实际情况写一份留学申请简历或一份求职简历。

第二章　医用信函

第一节　医用信函的主要内容

1.1　定义

医用信函是指医学工作者在医疗、科研和教育活动中所书写的信函。通常分为临床书信、科研书信和教育书信三大类。对医学生而言,最常接触到的英文书信是科研书信。

科研书信是医学生或医务人员向学校、科研机构、基金会、学术期刊、合作研究团队等发送的信函,用于申请留学或课题研究资金、提交研究报告、寻求合作等。最常见的包括申请信、推荐信、投稿信、邀请信等。

随着网络通信软件、数字媒体等现代交流方式的迅速发展,信函大多以电子邮件的形式传递和交流。

1.2　信函格式

医用科研书信的格式通常包括以下几个部分。

(1)信头(Heading):信头部分包括信函的日期、信纸上方的发件人和收件人的姓名、职称、机构地址等信息。发件人的信息通常写在信纸或电子邮件的右上角,收件人的信息写在发件人信息下一两行的左上角。一般给比较生疏的朋友写信或者是公事信函,需要写上详细的信息,而熟悉的朋友之间可以省略。常规的顺序是先写地址再写日期,地址从小到大,先写门牌号、路号,再写区名、市名、省名,最后写国名。

(2)称呼(Salutation):应根据收件人的身份和职称使用准确而礼貌的称谓,如"Dear Professor Smith"。常用在收件人名字前的尊称有:Mr. 、Mrs. 、Miss、Professor(Prof.)、Dr. 等。给机构写信,或者不知道收件人是谁时,常用"To whom it may concern",即"致有关人士"。

(3)信函正文(Body):正文分为引言、主体和结尾三个部分。引言应简单明了地表达写信目的;主体部分详细介绍请求、建议、共享的内容,结合文献或数据提供支持证据;结尾部分礼貌地表示感谢并期待对方的回复或进一步合作。

（4）结尾问候(Closure)：信末应以礼貌而恰当的方式结束,如祝愿对方身体健康、事事顺利等。例如：I am looking forward to hearing from you. 盼早日回信。With best regards. 祝好。Thank you for your help! 感谢你的帮助!

（5）署名(Signature)：在信末署名,并附上发件人的姓名、职务和联系方式。署名前一般会加上 Yours sincerely、Yours truly、Yours faithfully、Most sincerely、Faithfully yours 等作为结束语。

1.3 书写要求

撰写科研书信,要注意态度礼貌、诚挚、谦逊,尊重收信人的身份和职务,尊重对方国家的交流方式和规范。行文要逻辑清晰,层次分明,便于读者理解。在字数有限的情况下,要尽可能简洁、明了地表达自己的目的和需求。在信中陈述研究或调研的真实情况和需求,实事求是,不夸大其词。

科研信函的语法特点与正式文书相似,应使用正确的格式、词汇和语法,注意使用专业术语,避免使用过于口语化的词汇或表达方式。科研信函常用被动语态表达自己的观点、意愿或建议,以显得客观中立。

第二节　举例说明

2.1 申请信

2.1.1 定义

申请信(Application letter)是一种用英语书写的正式信件,用于向学术机构、教育机构、公司或其他相关机构提出申请,表达求职、申请学位、奖学金等事项。它通常包含向收件人介绍自己,说明申请事项的目的,并陈述申请的原因和背景。申请信是申请材料中非常重要的一部分,一封好的申请信,能够帮助申请者在众多申请者中脱颖而出,因此申请信的撰写尤为重要。

撰写申请信之前,申请者需要了解目标学校和导师的研究方向、课程设置、招生要求等信息,以便更好地准备申请材料。申请信不是论文,不需要使用太多的学术术语和复杂的句式,要用简短、有力的语言表达自己的观点和想法。信中要突出自己的优势和与申请相关的经验,并提供相关证明材料。申请信还应该注意书信格式和礼仪,注意语法、拼写和标点符号的正确性,以展示申请者的专业素质和语言能力。

2.1.2 格式和内容

（1）开头部分　需要写上自己的联系方式和日期,然后写上收信人的姓名和地址。

（2）正文部分

• 简要介绍自己，并表达申请的原因以及申请的兴趣和动机。例如，介绍自己目前的学习情况、教育背景、申请的项目/奖学金；表达对学校或导师的认可和申请意愿；可以介绍自己为什么选择该学校、该导师，以及希望在该学校或导师下进行何种研究。

• 详细说明自己的研究方向和兴趣。可以介绍自己在某个领域的研究成果或经验，一些与申请相关的成就和特长，以及对该领域未来发展的看法和期望。注意，要把自己重要的优势和成就突出展现，同时要避免重复和冗长。

• 谈谈自己的学业规划和未来发展。可以介绍自己的学业目标和计划，以及如何利用该学校或导师的资源实现自己的目标；强调自己愿意为该机构或项目的发展做出贡献，并提供一些具体的想法或计划。

（3）结尾部分要表达感谢并提供联系方式。使用正式结束语，如"best/kind regards"等，并在下方注明姓名、学术职位、机构和联系方式。

2.1.3 英文申请信常用句型

• I am writing to apply for admission to your esteemed institution/program/scholarship.

• I am highly interested in pursuing further studies in ...

• My strong academic background has equipped me with a solid foundation in ...

• I am confident that my qualifications align with the requirements of this position.

• The comprehensive curriculum and cutting-edge research facilities offered by ABC Medical School align perfectly with my academic and career goals.

• I am deeply motivated to pursue further studies in pharmacology under the supervision of Prof. ...

• I have a strong academic background in ...

• I am confident that I would be a valuable asset to your organization.

• I would greatly appreciate the opportunity to discuss my application further.

• I am available for an interview at your convenience.

• I have attached my resume for your review.

• Thank you for considering my application.

Application for the doctoral program

Zhou Xiaolong

School of Clinical Medicine

Southern Medical University

Guangdong Province

P. R. China

E-mail: XiaolongZhou@xxxx.com

Mobile: +86 137-12345678

September 1, 2023

Dear Prof. Alan,

I am writing to apply for the doctoral program at your esteemed institution. I am highly interested in the excellent medical education and research opportunities your university offers, and I aspire to be a part of your institution.

Currently, I am a medical student at Southern Medical University. Throughout my medical studies, I have gained a wide range of medical knowledge and accumulated extensive clinical experience through internships and practical training. I have a particular interest in Pediatrics and have some research experience in this field.

Over the past two years, I have interned at the Pediatrics department of a large hospital, where I collaborated with a mentor on a research project related to childhood pneumonia. Our research findings were published in an international medical journal and received recognition from peers in the field. This project allowed me to gain a deeper understanding of the research process and scientific methods, as well ashoned my analytical and problem-solving skills.

I believe that under the nurturing of the doctoral program at your institution, I can further enhance my research abilities and make contributions to addressing significant medical issues. I am eager to collaborate with the faculty team at your university to delve into and expand my knowledge in the field of Pediatrics.

Attached please find my resume and recommendation letters for your review. Should you require any additional materials or have any questions, I would be more than willing to provide them. I sincerely hope to have the opportunity to be a part of your doctoral program and will exert my utmost effort to contribute to it. Thank you very much for considering my application. I look forward to your favorable response.

Best regards,
Zhou Xiaolong

2.2 推荐信

2.2.1 定义

推荐信(Reference letter/Recommendation letter)是在申请过程中,由推荐人为受推荐人向其将要申请的学校或机构撰写的信件。在医学院校硕士或博士的英文申请中,推荐信对于申请人来说非常重要,因为它可以提供对申请人能力和素质的官方认可和担保。

招生官除了阅读申请者的标化成绩、GPA和陈述性文书外,还需要一份从第三方来的信息,以验证申请者的科研能力和水平,同时让招生委员从客观角度了解个人特质。因此,精心撰写的推荐信可以有效地将学生与其他申请人区分开来,并为他们的性格、职业道德,以及在高等教育中取得成功的潜力提供独特的视角。

2.2.2 格式和内容

(1)开头部分
推荐信的开头应该简洁明了,包含写信人的联系方式以及被推荐人的姓名和申请的学位。
(2)正文部分
• 简要介绍推荐人与被推荐人的关系,包括任课教师、导师或研究合作伙伴等。如果推荐人职位高,其推荐信也会有更大的影响力。
• 重点描述被推荐人的学术能力、研究经验和专业知识,在医学领域中的表现以及对医学及相关科目的热诚和动力。可以列举一些实例来支持对被推荐人的评价。
• 阐述被推荐人的个性特质、领导才能、沟通技巧和团队协作精神等,还可以通过一些实例来支持对被推荐人个性特质的评价。
(3)结尾部分
结束时,推荐人应该总结对被推荐人的评价,并强调被推荐人对于医学领域的承诺和自我提升的潜力。同时,推荐人也可以表示对被推荐人未来发展的期望,并愿意提供进一步信息和支持。

2.2.3 英文推荐信常用句型

• I am pleased to recommend her to ...

- I have had the pleasure of knowing her for two years and can confidently attest to her exceptional qualities.

- His dedication, intelligence, and strong work ethic make him an ideal candidate for … .

- I have been consistently impressed with his ability to … .

- He is a natural leader who can effectively motivate and inspire others.

- His strong analytical and problem-solving skills allow him to excel in any situation.

- He consistently goes above and beyond expectations and is always willing to take on additional responsibilities.

- He is a team player who collaborates well with others, contributing to a positive and productive working environment.

- I wholeheartedly recommend … and am confident that he will excel in his future endeavors.

- Please do not hesitate to contact me with further questions.

2.2.4 示例

Reference Letter

Prof. Guofeng Wang

Department of Pharmacy

Anhui Medical University

No. 81 Meishan Road Hefei China

Anhui Province,P. R. China

(+86)0551—6516xxxx

22-10-2023

Prof. Lawrence Cooper

935Rator Street

Santa Rosa MN 98804

Dear Prof. Cooper,

　　I am writing to highly recommend Ms. Yang Li as a candidate for your Ph. D. program in Pharmaceutics. I am her former supervisor at Anhui Medical University, China, and had the opportunity to work with her closely on her graduation thesis.

During the year that Ms. Li was associated with me on a project to develop a sustained release preparation for a compound herbal medicine, she impressed me with her enthusiasm, resourcefulness, and creativity. She approached the challenging task with determination and tackled the volatile nature of the compound substances with ease, assuming a key role in our research team. Her dedication to the project and ability to find innovative solutions to technical difficulties was remarkable.

Throughout our collaboration, Ms. Li has demonstrated exceptional scientific rigor and a bold spirit of adventure in her approach to research. She has a strong educational background and has shown a remarkable ability in laboratory experimentation. Her proficiency in English, an uncommon skill among her peers, has enabled her to read professional journals and documents with ease and engage in fruitful discussions with native English speakers.

As her teacher and former supervisor, I am immensely proud of Ms. Li's academic achievements. She has demonstrated great potential and is an outspoken standout among her peers. In my opinion, the pursuit of a graduate degree in Pharmaceutics in a technologically advanced country would greatly enrich Ms. Li's development and push her to the forefront of her field. I have no doubt that she would make the most of this opportunity and emerge as a leading pharmacist.

Finally, I would like to reiterate my strong recommendation of Ms. Yang Li as a highly deserving candidate for your Ph. D. program. Her academic excellence and positive personality make her an excellent choice for this opportunity.

Yours Sincerely
Prof. Guofeng Wang

2.3 投稿信

2.3.1 定义

投稿信(Cover letter)是指研究者向医学类学术期刊投稿时所写的信函,用于向编辑部提交研究论文的意向并对研究内容、方法和结果进行简要介绍。投稿信是编辑对论文的第一印象,也是初步评判论文是否可以被期刊接收的重要依据,因此投稿信的撰写是非常重要的。

在写投稿信之前,要仔细阅读目标期刊的投稿指南和要求,写作语言简练明确,突出研究亮点和创新,避免使用夸张的措辞或庸俗的形容词。按照结构要求将信件分为引言、研究内容、重要性和创新性等部分。

2.3.2 格式和内容

（1）开头部分

投稿信的开头应该包括研究者的联系信息,如姓名、机构、地址、电话、电子邮件等,信件编写的日期,编辑的姓名和学术期刊的名称及地址,及对编辑的尊称,如"Dear Dr. XX"。

（2）正文部分

• 介绍自己,重点介绍自己的研究领域和研究经验,并表达对该期刊的兴趣等。

• 简要介绍研究的目的、方法、结果和主要发现等。

• 说明为何该期刊的读者会对这项研究感兴趣,研究的重要性和创新性,研究结果对这个领域的重要性等。

• 最后说明作者需要遵守的特定要求（例如伦理标准）。

（3）结尾部分

感谢编辑的时间和关注并表达期望与期刊合作的愿望;适用的正式结束语,如"Sincerely"等;研究者签名,并在下方注明姓名、学术职位、机构和联系方式。

2.3.3 英文投稿信常用句型

• I am writing to submit my article/paper for consideration.

• I am very interested in publishing my work in your esteemed journal.

• I believe that my research findings are significant and relevant to the field.

• I have attached my manuscript for your review.

• I would greatly appreciate it if you could consider my submission for publication.

• I am willing to make any necessary revisions suggested by the reviewers.

• Thank you for your time and consideration.

• I look forward to hearing from you soon.

投稿信必须包含以下内容:

• We confirm that this manuscript has not been published elsewhere and is not under consideration by another journal.

• All authors have approved the manuscript and agree with its submission to ...

2.3.4 示例

Dr. Smith White

Editor-in-Chief

Journal of Chronic Disease Treatment

May 15，2023

Dear Dr. Smith，

We are submitting our article "Exercise Intervention: Mental Health Impact and Chronic Disease Management" for consideration as a regular research article in the *Journal of Chronic Disease Treatment*.

In our previous work (Tan et al. , 2022), we showed that a treatment X was more effective than a treatment Y in reducing a specific chronic disease Z. However，we observed that both treatments were more effective during the winter months compared to the summer. To explore this observation，we conducted additional research，which we describe in the current article.

We found that temperature did not impact the effectiveness of either treatment on disease Z. However，through detailed analysis of patient behavior，we determined that patients were more likely to be away from home during the summer and therefore more likely to miss their medication. By implementing a dosing strategy to minimize this effect，we were able to detect no significant difference between summer and winter effectiveness of either treatment.

We believe that this article will be of interest to your readers as it not only demonstrates increased treatment effectiveness without increasing overall dosage，but also highlights interesting aspects of patient behavior that have gained attention in chronic disease treatment over the past decade.

We confirm on behalf of all the authors of this article that no author has any conflict of interest to disclose，all authors have approved the version submitted for publication，the work in this article is original and has not been published previously，and the article is not under consideration by any other journal.

We appreciate your time and consideration of our manuscript. If any further information is required，please do not hesitate to contact us directly. We look forward to hearing from you.

Yours sincerely,
Dr. Junjie Tan

Department of Nutrition Sciences
Beijing University Health Science Center
38Xueyuan Rd ，Haidian District，Beijing，China
Email：TJJ@bjmu.edu
Phone：（086）010-8280××××

2.4 邀请信

2.4.1 定义

邀请信(Invitation letter)是由主办单位或会议组委会代表向受邀嘉宾发出的信函,目的是邀请受邀嘉宾参加医学会议,分享专业知识和经验,促进医学领域的学术交流。

2.4.2 格式

英文医学会议邀请信通常包含以下几个部分:

(1) 开头部分

包含主办单位或会议组委会的名称、地址、联系方式等信息;发信日期;收信人信息,包括姓名、职务、单位、地址等;称呼:以尊敬的方式称呼被邀请嘉宾。

(2) 正文部分

• 明确邀请的目的,例如邀请演讲、主持、展示研究成果等;

• 用简洁明了的语言描述会议的重要性、议题和邀请嘉宾的特点;

• 提供详细的会议时间、地点、议程等信息以便受邀嘉宾做出安排;

• 以礼貌和尊重的语气表达邀请,并表示期待对方的出席;

• 附带会议的议程、背景资料或其他相关材料,以便受邀嘉宾更好地了解会议内容。

(3) 结尾部分

表达诚挚的邀请和期待收到回复的愿望;署名,会议主办单位或组委会代表的姓名和职务。

2.4.3 英文邀请信常用句型

• We cordially invite you to attend our event.

• We are pleased to invite you to attend our upcoming medical conference.

• We cordially invite you to be a keynote speaker at the medical congress that will be held on ...

- We kindly request your presence at the medical forum, where you will have the opportunity to share your insights and experiences with fellow medical professionals.

- Your contribution as a distinguished guest at the medical convention would greatly enhance the quality of the event.

- We hope that you will be able to join us at the medical seminar, where you can share your valuable insights and contribute to the advancement of medical knowledge.

- We kindly request your presence at the medical summit, where you can engage in fruitful exchanges with colleagues and foster collaborations.

- The conference aims to provide a platform for healthcare professionals to exchange knowledge, share experiences, and network with each other.

- We kindly request you to confirm your attendance and let us know if you require any further information or assistance.

- Thank you for your attention, and we hope to see you at the conference.

2.4.4 示例

Dear Professor,

We are delighted to invite you to the International Conference on Clinical Medicine, which will take place on September 9 at XYZ Medical University. This conference aims to bring together esteemed medical professionals, researchers, and experts from around the world to share their knowledge, advancements, and experiences in the field of clinical medicine.

The conference will provide a platform for in-depth discussions on various topics, including but not limited to clinical research, disease management, diagnostic techniques, therapeutic interventions, and healthcare innovations. Renowned keynote speakers will be delivering enlightening presentations, and there will be interactive sessions, poster presentations, and networking opportunities for participants to engage in fruitful exchanges of ideas and foster collaborations. We believe that your expertise and contributions would greatly enhance the conference. Therefore, we cordially invite you to attend and present your research findings, clinical case studies, or innovative approaches related to clinical medicine. Your valuable insights will undoubtedly contribute to the success of the conference and further advancements in the field of clinical medicine. find attached the conference brochure, which contains comprehensive information about the conference agenda, registration procedures, and guidelines for abstract submission.

We kindly request you to submit your abstract by July 18th for consideration. Early bird registration is available until June 30th, ensuring discounted rates for participants. Should you have any queries or require further information, please do not hesitate to contact our conference secretariat at ICCM@xyzmu.edu.cn. We will be more than happy to assist you with any concerns. We look forward to your presence at the International Conference on Clinical Medicine and the opportunity to interact with you and learn from your expertise. Your participation will undoubtedly contribute to the success of the conference and the advancement of clinical medicine. Thank you for your attention, and we hope to see you at the conference.

Sincerely Yours,

Linda Yeung

Organizing Committee of International Conference on Clinical Medicine

220 Handan Rd, Fudan University, Shanghai, China

Email: admin@fdu.edu

Tel：086-123-456789

第三节　练习巩固

1. 请翻译下面的句子。

（1）我对神经外科学非常感兴趣，想向贵校争取录取机会。

（2）我确信我的资历符合这个奖学金的要求，我期待着能够成为贵校的一员。

（3）我在肿瘤学方面有坚实的学术背景，这让我具备了进一步研究的基础。

（4）非常感激您能考虑我的申请，我对在史密斯教授的指导下进行进一步的学习充满了热情。

2. 将下面的句子补充完整。

（1）I am writing to ＿＿＿＿＿＿＿＿＿＿（强烈推荐）him as a potential candidate for your esteemed institution.

（2）It is with the greatest pleasure that I recommend Meimei Han for the ＿＿＿＿＿＿＿＿（奖学金）you have available.

（3）Based on his ＿＿＿＿＿＿＿＿（突出表现）and exceptional abilities, I am confident that he will make a valuable contribution to your program.

（4）She has demonstrated exceptional leadership a ＿＿＿＿＿＿＿＿（团队建设技巧），

making her a standout candidate in any field.

(5) I am writing to express my support for his _____ (职位申请)，as he has excelled in all aspects of the selection criteria.

3. 选择合适的单词填空。

esteemed	approved	field	manuscript	publication
consideration	hearing	attached	reviewers	article

(1) I am writing to submit my _____ for consideration.

(2) I am very interested in publishing my work in your _____ journal.

(3) I believe that my research findings are significant and relevant to the _____.

(4) I have _____ my manuscript for your review.

(5) I would greatly appreciate it if you could consider my submission for _____.

(6) I am willing to make any necessary revisions suggested by the _____.

(7) Thank you for your time and _____.

(8) I look forward to _____ from you soon.

(9) We confirm that this _____ has not been published elsewhere and is not under consideration by another journal.

(10) All authors have _____ the submission and agree with its submission to your journal.

4. 翻译句子中画线的部分。

(1) The lead researcher of the medical conference will give a keynote speech on the topic "Prevention and treatment of Disease".

_____

(2) The goals of the medical conference are designed to improve the health outcomes of patients.

_____

(3) The medical conference will provide an opportunity for attendees to network and share ideas with other top medical professionals.

_____

(4) The brochure of the medical conference is available in the attached PDF file.

_____

(5) We look forward to your participation in one of the exciting panel discussions in the medical conference.

_____

第三章　医学病历

第一节　病历的基本要求和内容

1.1　定义

病历是指医务人员在医疗活动过程中形成的文字、符号、图表和影像等资料的总和。病历书写是指医务人员通过问诊、查体、辅助检查、诊断、治疗、护理等医疗活动获得有关资料，并进行归纳、分析、整理形成医疗活动记录的行为。

病历既是诊治疾病的重要依据，也是医学科研的重要资料。同时，它还是具有法律效力的证据。因此，临床医生书写病历，应当客观、真实、准确、完整、规范。

1.2　书写病历的基本要求

（1）记载真实，书写规范，内容完整，语言简练，标点正确，字迹清晰。

（2）时间采用 24 小时制的国际记录方式。如：2022 年 3 月 15 日下午一点半，应写为：03 - 15 - 2022,13:30。

（3）症状、体征、病名、身体器官等用医学英语术语表述。

（4）记载病人过敏的药物，且做明显标志，以引起有关人员注意。

（5）严格遵守所在国家、医院对病历书写的各项规定。

1.3　病历的基本内容

国际上对病历内容的格式没有统一要求，一份完整的住院病历，主要内容如下：

- 一般资料（General Data）
- 主诉（Chief Complaints）
- 现病史（Present Illness）
- 既往病史（Past Medical History）
- 个人史（Social History）
- 家族史（Family Medical History）

- 系统回顾（System Review）
- 体格检查（Physical Examination）
- 过敏史（Allergies）
- 曾用药物（Medications）
- 化验室检查（Laboratory Data）
- 印象/初步诊断（Impression/Tentative Diagnosis）

具体的病历报告可根据实际情况合并或者删减内容。

第二节　举例说明

2.1　一般资料（General Data）

一般资料包括病历号（Case Number）；姓名（Name）；性别（Sex），填写男（Male）或女（Female）；年龄（Age），填写周岁年龄；种族或民族（Race）；出生日期（Birth Date）；出生地（Birth Place）；婚姻状况（Marital Status），未婚填写 Single 或 Unmarried，已婚填写 Married；职业（Occupation）；住址（Address）；入院时间（Admission Data）；记录日期（Record Data）；主诉可靠程度（Reliability），通常填写"可靠"（Reliable），"不太确定"（Uncertain）或"混乱"（Confused）。与此相关的还有一栏是供史者（Complainer of History），可根据实际填写 Patient、Husband、Wife、Son、Father 等。

其他内容，如手机号码、家庭地址等可根据实际需要判断是否需要填写。

一般资料，可以以几种形式出现在病历上，大多是在病历的首页印好了有关表格，让患者自行填写。如下表所示：

Medical No.：756943	
Name：Yue Jun-rong	**Sex**：Female
Age：42	**Date of birth**：07-27-1981
Marital status：Married	**Nationality**：Han
Occupation：Unemployment	**Phone No.**：12345678901
Address：Xiaochang county of Xiaogan city in Hubei	
Reliability：Reliable	**Complainer**：Patient
Patient condition：Fair	**Date of record**：02-27-2021

把上述资料并入病历首段，可以写为：

The patient，a 42-year-old female，unemployed，was first seen in the office with a complaint of 3 days' severe cough.

患者是一个 42 岁的无业女性，首次就诊，主诉为严重咳嗽三天。

2.2　主诉 (Chief Complaints)

　　主诉应客观反映病人诉说的相关症状,首先要真实,其次文字要简明,有概括性。主要症状一般不超过 3 个,并说明各自持续的时间。主诉可使用省略句或短语表达。

2.2.1　常见症状

abdominal pain 腹痛	asthma 哮喘
poor appetite 胃口差	burning pain 灼痛
black tarry stools 黑色柏油便	constipation 便秘
diarrhea 腹泻	polyuria 多尿
dizziness 眩晕	dull ache 钝痛
dyspnea 呼吸困难	dyspepsia 消化不良
edema 水肿	epigastric pain 上腹痛
heavy menstruation 月经过多	fatigue 疲劳
fever 发热	frequent maturation 月经不调
heartburn 胃灼热	hemafecia 便血
insomnia 失眠	jaundice 黄疸
lethargic 嗜睡	melena 黑便
nasal obstruction 鼻塞	nausea 恶心
oliguria 少尿	obnubilation 神志不清
sore throat 喉咙痛	squeezing and crushing pain 挤压痛
stiff neck 落枕	stomachache 胃痛
vomiting 呕吐	

2.2.2　常见句式

　　• The patient was admitted with a chief complaint of vomiting and fever for 3 days.

　　• The patient complained chiefly of insomnia for a month.

　　• The patient presented a severe stomachache for a week.

　　• The patient entered the hospital with complaints of polyuria and edema for a week.

　　• The patient was referred to otolaryngology department because of painful swelling in the throat for a week.

2.2.3　示例

　　例 1:CHIEF COMPLAINT:right breast mass found for more than half a month.
　　主诉:发现右乳房肿块超过半个月。

例 2：CHIEF COMPLAINT：4-hour crushing retrosternal chest pain.

主诉：胸骨后挤压性疼痛 4 小时。

例 3：CHIEF COMPLAINT：This patient presented today complaining of burning pain when bending 1 hour after eating. She indicated the problem location was upper left stomach and severity of condition was worsening.

主诉：今日接诊病人主诉饭后一小时弯腰时左上胃灼痛，并且越来越严重。

2.3 现病史(Present Illness)

现病史是对主诉内容的进一步延伸。从医生的角度全面说明现有疾病的起病时间、症状的特点、发展过程、症状间关系、诊疗史、病人身体现状等。现病史作为病史的重要部分，应全面完整。

现病史的内容应按时间顺序组织。病人入院时自述情况一般用过去时或过去完成时。记录病人现状一般多用现在时或现在完成时。

2.3.1 常用词语

attack/onset 发病，发作   accidentally perceived 偶然察觉

abrupt attack 突然发作   acute 急性的

explosive 爆发的   persistent 持续的

focal 病灶的   afebrile 不发烧的

sequel 继发症   constitutional/general 全身性的

local 局部的   spastic 痉挛的

masked 隐蔽的   recurrent 反复不定的

relapsing 复发的   intermittent 间歇性的

be accompanied by 伴有   erupt simultaneously 并发

complication 并发症   premonitory symptom 先兆症状

asymptomatic 无症状的   persist 持续

worsen 恶化   have a relapse 复发

improve 改善   be relieved 缓解

aggravate 加剧   subside 减轻

2.3.2 常用句式

- The patient began having a mild fever a week ago.
- The patient had a sudden onset of angina in the heart.
- His illness was characterized by a high fever and persistent pain in the abdomen.
- The recurrent fever assumed the character of bronchitis.
- The patient was admitted without symptoms of fever or diarrhea.

- He <u>denied</u> hypertension or atherosclerosis.
- Such attacks usually <u>subsided promptly</u> after a rest.
- The pain was <u>intensified</u> when climbing the stairs.

2.3.3 示例

PRESENT ILLNESS：About 20 years ago，the patient suffered for the first time from palpitations which occurred after she had done vigorous physical exercise，and which have been gradually worsening ever since. Ten years ago，a cardiac murmur was discovered and a diagnosis of heart disease was given，which was not treated. Nevertheless，she had been capable of doing light work until half a month ago，when she caught a cold，which was accompanied by chills，cough non-productive of sputum. In the last few days，her condition has been aggravated by epigastric distention，nausea，vomiting and edema of the ankles；she is thus unable to lie supine. Palpitations and dyspnea are further aggravated at the same time.

现病史：患者20年前剧烈运动后首次出现心悸，此后症状逐渐恶化。10年前，查出心脏杂音，并被诊断为心脏病，未做治疗。此后仍可从事轻体力活动。半月前患重感冒，伴寒战，咳嗽无痰液。近几日病情加重，出现上腹胀气、恶心、呕吐和脚踝水肿，无法仰卧，心悸和呼吸困难进一步加剧。

2.4 既往病史(Past Medical History)

既往病史记录患者以往患过的疾病和治疗情况、预防接种、传染病等相关情况。如有过敏史，可用红笔或者其他特殊方式记下致敏药物或物质，引起相关人员注意。也可单独记录在后面的过敏史栏目中。

既往病史是记录病人过去病史的，所以时态常用一般过去时或过去完成时。也可使用省略句或者短语。例如：Healthy、no history of hypertension、no history of tuberculosis and radiation contact、no history of drug allergy。

2.4.1 常用词语

tuberculosis 肺结核	pneumonia 肺炎
allergy 过敏反应	cholera 霍乱
rheumatism 风湿	hepatitis B 乙肝
dysentery 痢疾	plague 瘟疫
influenza 流感	malaria 疟疾
tetanus 破伤风	mumps 腮腺炎
typhoid 伤寒	varicella 水痘
smallpox 天花	bronchitis 支气管炎

医学英语写作

2.4.2 常用句式

- The patient had been sound until two months ago when he had a severe chest pain.
- Past medical history included appendectomy in 2002 and tonsillectomy in 2018.
- He had a 3 months' history of chronic UTI.
- The patient was diagnosed with hepatitis A.
- The patient denied any history of heart attack.
- He was inoculated with hepatitis B virus at age 4.

2.4.3 示例

PAST MEDICAL HISTORY：The patient had a history of myelodysplastic syndrome，hypertension，and coronary artery disease for which he had a four-vessel coronary artery bypass 2 years prior to admission. The patient had no known history of diabetes.

既往病史：患者有骨髓增生异常综合征、高血压和冠心病病史。入院前2年曾接受四支冠状动脉搭桥术。患者不知晓糖尿病病史。

2.5 个人史(Social History)

个人史记录病人的个体情况。主要包括：① 患者的生活及嗜好,如吸烟、喝酒或吸毒的习惯;② 职业和工作环境;③ 婚姻及生育;④ 月经(此项针对成年女性);⑤ 小儿个人史(此项针对幼儿),如:自然产或剖宫产、母乳或配方奶、发育和预防接种等。

2.5.1 常用词语

drugs 毒品

chronic alcoholism 慢性酒精中毒

a heavy smoker 有烟瘾的人

condom 安全套

infertility 不孕

deformity 畸形

abortion/miscarriage 流产

leucorrhea 白带

irregular menstruation 月经不调

hard liquor/spirits 烈酒

partiality for a kind of food 偏食

be indulged in drinking 纵酒

contraception 避孕

delivery/labour 分娩

intermarriage 近亲结婚

induced abortion 人工流产

amenorrhea 闭经

excessive menstruation 月经过多

2.5.2 示例

例 1：

SOCIAL HISTORY：The patient had smoked 1.5 packs of cigarettes per day for

51 years and had quit 3 years ago. He was retired from the advertising industry and admitted to occasional alcohol use.

个人史：患者每天吸烟1.5包,持续51年,3年前戒烟。他从广告行业退休,并承认偶尔饮酒。

例2：

SOCIAL HISTORY：The baby was born by caesarean birth. He has been basically fed by bottle because his mother has been unwell since his birth. His weight is far below the average.

个人史：患儿为剖宫产,基本为奶粉喂养,因为他的母亲从他出生后就身体不适。患儿体重远低于平均值。

2.6 家族病史(Family Medical History)

家族病史记录患者近亲(父母、兄弟姊妹、子女等)和配偶的健康情况,尤其是传染病和遗传病的相关情况。如有死亡,说明死亡原因和时间。

例：

FAMILY MEDICAL HISTORY：The patient's mother suffered from chronic pulmonary disease and died of pulmonary cancer three years ago. His brother has pneumonia. His father is healthy. There is a high incidence of lung disease in the family.

家族病史：患者母亲患有慢性肺病,三年前死于肺癌。患者哥哥目前感染肺炎。患者父亲健康。但家族中肺病的患病率高。

2.7 系统回顾(System Review)

系统回顾是对病人身体各个系统病情的详细列举。无论与现在/当前病症是否相关,无论结果是阴性还是阳性都要罗列。系统回顾一般用短语。

例1：

SYSTEM REVIEW

Neuromuscular：weakness of muscles.

Respiratory：dyspnea; coarse crackles; wheezes.

Digestive：nausea, vomits after eating.

例2：

SYSTEM REVIEW

Respiratory：No history of tachypnea.

Circulation：hypertension.

Bones and joints：Negative.

Endocrine：Non-contributory.

Digestive: Bowl movement abnormal for a week.

2.8　体格检查(Physical Examination)

医生通常会通过视、听、触、叩对病人进行检查,查找有关体征,并记录下来以支持正确的诊断。体格检查主要包括:一般资料(体温、脉搏、心率、血压、呼吸、发育)、皮肤黏膜、头颈、胸腹、泌尿生殖、四肢脊柱、神经反射等。

例1:

PHYSICAL EXAMINATON: Temperature: 37 ℃. Pulse: 95 times/min. He is well developed and moderately nourished. No pigmentation. No skin eruption. Spider angioma was not seen. No pitting edema. Superficial lymph nodes were not found enlarged in his neck.

体格检查:体温 37 ℃,脉搏 95 次/分钟。患者发育良好,营养适中。无色素沉着,无皮疹。蜘蛛血管瘤未见,点状水肿未见。颈部未发现浅表淋巴结肿大。

例2:

PHYSICAL EXAMINATION: Physical examination was unremarkable except for a thoracotomy scar in the left hemothorax, decreased breath sounds, and dullness to percussion of the left base. There was no hemoptysis.

体格检查:除了左半胸开胸术疤痕、呼吸音降低和左胸基部叩击音沉闷,体格检查无异常。没有咯血。

2.9　过敏史(Allergies)和曾用药物(Medications)

过敏史描述病人对某些药物或物质过敏的情况,如过敏史在既往病史中出现,此处可省略。曾用药物包括近期和当前服用的药物及使用剂量。两者常用简单句和省略句表达。

例:

ALLERGIES: allergy to aspirin resulting in rash and gastrointestinal upset.
MEDICATIONS: Penicillin as needed.

2.10　化验资料(Laboratory Data)

化验资料一般按以下顺序排列:基础化验室检查结果、专科化验室检查结果、影像学检查结果和心电图检查结果。

例1:

LAB DATA: Computerized tomography of the abdomen and pelvis was significant for acute pancreatitis without necrosis or abscess. No gallstones, strictures, or bile duct dilatation were visualized; bronchiectasis was present in the right middle lobe. Endoscopic ultrasound disclosed no abnormalities.

化验资料:腹部和骨盆计算机断层扫描结果显示未坏死或脓肿的急性胰腺炎。未发现胆结石、狭窄或胆管扩张。右肺中叶出现支气管扩张。超声内镜检查未发现异常。

例2:

LAB DATA: Laboratory tests were normal except for leukocytosis and elevated erythrocyte sedimentation rate (52 mm/hour). All biochemistry parameters including tumor markers were within the normal limits. The stool was positive for cysts of histolytica. Ultrasonography showed marked bowel wall thickness in the sigmoid-descending colon junction. Maximal wall thickness was 20mm.

化验资料:除了白细胞增多和红细胞沉降率升高(52毫米/时)外,实验室检查基本正常。包括肿瘤标志物在内的所有生物化学参数均在正常范围内。粪便中溶组织囊肿呈阳性。超声检查显示乙状结肠降结肠交界处有明显的肠壁增厚。最大壁厚为20毫米。

2.11 印象/初步诊断(Impression/Primary Diagnosis)

顾名思义,这是医生综合各种情况后得出的初步诊断。诊断结果通常用名词短语表示。

例:

IMPRESSION:

1. Second degree burns involving 30% of body surface area including mouth and neck.

2. Possible inhalation injury.

初步诊断:

1. 二度烧伤涉及30%的体表面积,包括口腔和颈部。

2. 可能有吸入性损伤。

第三节 练习巩固

1. 判读下列句子分别是属于医学病历的哪个部分。

(1) The patient, a 19-year-old college student, was diagnosed at the age of 13 with Crohn disease, a chronic inflammatory disease that can affect the entire gastrointestinal tract from mouth to anus.

(2) The patient was brought to the emergency room by ambulance with chest pain that radiated down his arm, dyspnea, and syncope. Shortly after his admission,

his heart rate deteriorated into full cardiac arrest.

(3) E. G. , a twenty year old girl, complained of pain in her head, back, chest, and leg. She also had numbness and tingling in her legs and feet. Other injuries included a cut on her face and on her right arm and an obvious deformity to both her shoulder and knee.

(4) An abdominal ultrasound demonstrated passive congestion of the liver, small bilateral pleural effusions, gallbladder sludge, and normal sized kidneys with slightly increased cortical echogenicity. Repeated laboratory tests showed a gradual increase in blood urea nitrogen and serum creatinine. His liver function test results also increased.

(5) Possible recurrence of ovarian cancer.

2. 请根据上下文用括号中词语的正确形式补充完成下列句子。

(1) Her ECG on _____ (admit) presented tachycardia with a rate of 123 bpm with inverted T waves. A murmur _____ (hear) at S1.

(2) The 52-year-old middle school teacher, had myelofibrosis that had been in remission for 10 years. She _____ (see) her hematologist regularly and _____ (have) routine blood testing since the age of 28.

(3) After several weeks of fatigue, idiopathic joint and muscle _____ (ache), _____ (weak) and a frightening episode of syncope, she was admitted into the hospital.

(4) After a regimen of high dose chemotherapy _____ (shrink) the fibers in her bone marrow and a splenectomy, the patient received a stem cell transplant. The stem cells were obtained from blood _____ (donate) by her brother.

(5) The patient entered the hospital with nausea and _____ (vomit), a high fever and _____ (continue) right upper quadrant and subscapular pain.

3. 请把下面的医学病历翻译成汉语,注意表达清晰、措辞专业。

Chief Complaint:

Repeated vomiting for more than 2 weeks, aggravated for 3 days.

Present Illness:

The patient had nausea and vomiting after the dinner for no reason. The vomitus was what he ate all day and it had no special smell or blood. After the vomiting, the nausea disappeared. It was fine when he drank water and the passage of gas by anus was normal. He had no fever, headache, diarrhea, chest pain, angina or abnormal feeling in the throat. The symptom occurred every other day, so the patient didn't go for medical care. 3 days ago, the symptom worsened. The vomitus was also what he ate in the day but with some yellowish fluids. The patient went to the local hospital for treatment but didn't have any improvement. Then he was admitted to the hospital as "unknown vomiting".

The patient has a 5 kilograms weight loss since the illness. The appetite is poor. The mental state is good. The urine is normal and the stool is good with normal properties.

Past Medical History:

The patient had chronic gastritis for many years and the abdominal pain was under control on medication. Last May, he had a successful thoracoscopic surgery because of "rupture of bulla". He denied any history of hypertension, diabetes, tuberculosis or other infectious diseases. He also denied any history of allergy to drugs or food and had no history of trauma or blood transfusion. His immunizations are up to date.

Social History:

The patient was born in the rural areas of Anhui Province and denies any history of contact with any infectious diseases in the epidemic area. He is a retired primary school teacher and has no special contact with any chemicals. He smokes a pack of cigarettes per day for 10 years and drinks a little alcohol every day for 15 years.

Family Medical History:

Married at the age of 23. Wife had history of pulmonary tuberculosis, which was cured five years ago. Parents and a girl aged 27 are all living and well.

Impression:

Intestinal obstruction, pyloric obstruction.

第四章　会议通知

本章我们主要讨论医学领域的会议通知,常见的有学术会议、医学研讨会、医学年会、学术研修等。

第一节　会议通知的组成部分和写作方法

参见具体例文:

Annual Meeting of the National Advisory General Medical Sciences Council

The meeting will be held as a virtual meeting and open to the public. as indicated below. Individuals who plan to view the virtual meeting and need special assistance, such as sign language interpretation or other reasonable accommodations, should submit a request using the following link: https://www. nigms. nih. gov/Pages/ContactUs. aspx at least 5 days prior to the event. The open session will also be videocast, closed captioned, and can be accessed from the NIH Videocasting and Podcasting website (http://videocast. nih. gov).

Name of Committee: National Advisory General Medical Sciences Council.

Date: September 7, 2023.

Open: 9:30 to 12:30

Agenda: For the discussion of program policies and issues; opening remarks; report of the Director, NIGMS; and other business of the Council.

Location: National Institutes of Health, Natcher Building, Bethesda, MD 20892 (Virtual Meeting).

Closed: 13:30 to 16:30

Contact Person: Erica L. Brown, Ph. D. , Director, Division of Extramural Activities, National Institute of General Medical Sciences, National Institutes of Health, Natcher Building, Room 2AN24C, Bethesda, MD 20892, 301 - 594 - 4499, erica. brown@nih. gov.

Information is also available on the Institute's/Center's home page, http://www. nigms. nih. gov/About/Council, where an agenda and any additional information for the meeting will be posted when available.

(Catalogue of Federal Domestic Assistance Program No. 93. 859，Biomedical Research and Research Training，National Institutes of Health，HHS)

Date：June 27，2023.

Miguelina Perez,

Program Analyst，Office of Federal Advisory Committee Policy

根据以上例文,我们可以简单地把会议通知的构成要素概括如下:

会议标题

一、会议目的(Purpose)

二、与会人员(Participants)

三、会议时间(Date)

四、会议地点(Location)

五、会议日程(Agenda)

六、报到须知(Registration)

七、联系方式(Contacts)

当然,在具体的通知写作中,在此基础上,会产生各种变体,很多会议鼓励参会人员投稿,并发表相关论文,那么在通知中也应加上 Call for papers 和 Presentation 部分。但不论如何,会议通知的主要构成要素不能变,大致顺序也不变。

会议通知的写作要求如下:

(1)标题和目的要简单明了。目的是为了说明文件下发的合法性,增强文件的权威性,让参会单位和人员提高认识,引起重视,便于更好地落实。

(2)须知事项要明确。也就是说这个部分的写作最好要分条列项,逐项表述;做到简单、明了、具体;让人看后一目了然,没有歧义。

(3)要求部分要细致。在会议通知中,一定要把会议议题、参会人员、时间、地点、对与会者的要求(如是否需要论文投稿,会费和住宿交通费用等)一一交代清楚。

这些方面若能处理得当,就能使会议通知简明扼要、重点突出,且便于他人更好地知晓和办理。

第二节　练习巩固

根据下面材料,按照通知的写作要求,补充必要的素材,拟写一份会议通知。

中国生物医学工程大会暨创新医疗峰会决定于 2023 年 5 月 18 日至 21 日在江苏省苏州市召开,所属各单位均可派会员代表参加,规模适当控制。会议通知于 2 月 16 日发出。会议的内容是推进学科发展与产业融合,展现本领域科研新成果和新进展。报到和开会地点都是苏州金鸡湖国际会议中心。鼓励与会者撰写相关学术论文,带到会上交流,会前把稿子提前发到会务组。会务费自理。会议相关信息可与会务组联系。

第五章　学术报告

　　学术报告是国际学术会议的主要议程和主体内容,包括特邀报告、口头报告、张贴报告等形式,特邀报告又可分为主会场的大会报告和分会场的专题报告。大会报告多安排在开幕式之后,按其重要性及报告者的学术影响力确定报告的顺序。其中最为重要的大会报告被称为大会主旨报告(Keynote Speech),一般是相关研究领域内领衔的专家就学科或研究领域的热点、难点以及前沿问题做的报告。分会场的专题报告一般由会议主办机构直接指定并约稿。学术报告的水平在一定程度上体现了国际学术会议的水准,学术报告的学术价值和创新水平也决定了国际学术会议的影响力。

　　学术报告虽属于口语语体,但必须使用规范和正式的语言。学术报告要求内容专业、陈述直接、观点明确,对于报告者而言,对口头汇报的设计形式和报告时间的把握也非常重要。

第一节　学术报告常用语示例

　　英文口头学术报告的常用语很多,句法灵活多变。典型的学术报告用语包括导言和结束语、内容与致谢语,以及提问与答复语,熟练掌握这些语句有助于医务工作者在国际会议上顺利进行学术交流。

1.1　导言

　　学术报告的开场白很重要。宣读论文者可采用开门见山、致谢赞扬、介绍说明、风趣幽默、即席发挥等方法致开场白。

　　(1) Mr. Chairman, ladies and gentlemen, the title of my presentation is …

　　(2) Mr. Chairman, representatives, I am very glad to have the opportunity to report my research on such an occasion. I'll lay my stress on the following four aspects. The first aspect is …

　　(3) Thank you, Mr. Chairman. Ladies and gentlemen, what I am going to say can be roughly summed up into the following three points. First, let's see slide No. 1. (Turning to the slide projector)

　　(4) I work for … I have conducted research on … for over twenty years.

(5) Good afternoon, ladies and gentlemen, I have talked about my own work this morning, and now, with the kind permission of Mr. Chairman, I'll present the following paper for my colleague, Mr. ... who is unable to come. ...

(6) Good afternoon, everyone. There is a Chinese saying "with a hare under one's garment", to describe the uneasiness for a nervous person. That is how I am feeling at such a moment, and before such a big audience, as if I had a "hare under my garment".

Well, now, speaking about "nervous", I would like to show you the result of my experiment on the nervous system of a rabbit ...

1.2 结束语

学术报告常以直截了当、总结归纳和征询意见等方式结束。学术报告的结束语比较简单，一般是对听众的认真听讲表示感谢，有时还会再次总结所讲要点，或者表示希望听众对论文报告提出具体意见等。

(1) ... That's all. Thank you, Mr. Chairman. Thank you all.

(2) ... Well, I think this might be a good place for me to wind up my talk. Thank you everyone.

(3) ... The themes I have dealt with can be boiled down as follows: First,... ; second,... ; and last but not the least,... That's all for my talk. Thank you for your attention.

(4) ... In case I have made any careless mistakes and in order to clarify what I have said, let me just go over the main points again ... That's all. Thank you, everyone.

(5) ... That's all for my talk. Please don't hesitate to put forward your suggestions and advice, if you have any. Thank you.

1.3 内容语

学术报告通常由开头、展开和结尾三部分构成。展开部分的核心是传播信息、展示成果和沟通思想。展开部分除了要体现新颖丰富的报告内容外，还要展示文字组织的逻辑性，以及连贯、生动的表达。综合运用多种语言技巧，才能提高学术报告的实际效果。

(1) In our paper, we proposed a new method/novel structure ...

(2) The design of the experiment was to reveal ...

(3) According to this theory, we can obtain that ...

(4) The most important results are as follows ...

(5) As shown in Fig 1, we can see that ...

(6) It is a well-known fact that ...

(7) As far as we know/I am disposed to think that，...

(8) Let us have a closer look at ...

(9) Let me cite an example of ...

(10) It should be mentioned/pointed out that ...

(11) Let us consider what happens if ...

(12) The author introduces the new concept of ...

(13) ... In our early experiment，we inserted a temperature-controlled rubidium 87 filtering cell between the pumping lamp and the resonance cell. They are，er，well, something like two separated bulbs.

(14) In the experiment I discovered a new way，or rather I used a new method to observe the morphological changes.

(15) ... The next point is ... um，well. That is what we have done. Under that condition，which is essential for solving the problem，you know，I would say，we'll carefully perform the experiment. All right，here we are. The next point is ...

1.4 致谢语

学术报告中的致谢语用来表达对所有合作者劳动的尊重,致谢提供的信息对于听众判断报告的写作过程和价值也有一定的参考作用。致谢词要求态度端正,措辞恰如其分。

(1) This paper would not have been presented if I had not received the encouragement of ... and the beneficial discussions with ...

(2) These works are supported by the Science Foundation ... under the grant No. ... and the project under the No. ...

1.5 提问语

学术报告中的提问不同于一般交谈中的提问,具有即席答辩的性质。提问的目的因人因时而异。提问在学术报告的交流互动中起着主导作用。

(1) I don't quite understand what you really mean by saying ... Can you explain it again?

(2) I'm very keen on ... Would you please say a few more words about ... ?

(3) If I am not mistaken，you said ... As far as I know，however，... Would you please give us some explanations about this?

(4) I've got some insights from your views. But as to your sayings about ... I'm afraid at least ... Can I have your comments on that?

(5) Can I have a copy of your report on ... ?

1.6　答复语

　　学术报告的答复语是对提问语的反馈,讨论问答环节虽然时间不长,答复语也很短,但能集中反映出回答者在专业知识、语言能力、策略水平、临场经验等方面的情况。对于一般性提问,可以针对问题简明扼要予以答复。对于异议性问题,应尊重事实,阐明观点,以理服人。而对于带有指责意味的问题,更应小心谨慎,区别不同情况来处理。尤其注意在某些时候,需要运用委婉回避的语言策略,视具体情况灵活处理。

　　(1) To answer your question, I'll just repeat what I have said in my lecture ...

　　(2) If you're interested in the detailed parameters, I would suggest you look them up in the handout on Page 12, as has been shown in my presentation.

　　(3) To the best of my knowledge, you were asking me about ...

　　(4) One of the questions you put forward is about ... which I think, is very interesting. And now I'd like to answer the question as the following.

　　(5) Personally, I suppose/guess/think we're very likely to get more desirable results if we continue the treatment.

　　(6) I should have thought you misunderstood some of what I said in my lecture just now.

　　(7) A good point. Now I'll add something more to that ... as has been shown in the last slide.

　　(8) I appreciate your question. I'm afraid that our different views on the point may come from the different angles ... on the basis of the following three aspects: the first point is ...

　　(9) I don't like but I have to say it's ... I don't think it is helpful ... I'm afraid it's not within the area of this speech session.

　　(10) Thank you. As I said in my presentation, we haven't yet finalized the results of ... So I'm afraid it's a bit difficult for me to ... and I would like to inform you of ...

第二节　错例分析

2.1　书面语和口语的混用

例1:

Conclusions: Chronic hepatitis B virus infection, which usually starts in early childhood in China, seems lead not only to a greatly increased risk of death from liver disease but also to a somewhat lower cholesterol concentration in adulthood.

【分析】这段结论如出现在论文写作中,表达尚属清晰,但是用在学术报告中则显得冗长。本处可将书面语中常出现的复合句拆为口语中更为适用的简单句,使报告清晰有力。另外,一些书面语中较长的词组在口头报告中也可用一个词来替代,比如:has the capability 替换为 can;in view of the foregoing circumstances 替换为 therefore;due to the fact that 替换为 because;at this point in time 替换为 now,等等。

【修改】Conclusions:Chronic hepatitis B virus infection usually starts in early childhood in China. It seems lead not only to a greatly increased risk of death from liver disease but also to a somewhat lower cholesterol concentration in adulthood.

2.2 语言表达冗长,引导式和评价式结构过多

例 2:

It is well known that certain biological changes associated with depression may lead to dementia.

【分析】虽然学术报告形式上是口语体,但不能像日常生活中说话般随意,如引导式和评价式的结构基本可省略,直接讲述其后的主要观点,比如:There are many papers stating … /It is pointed out that … /Evidence has been presented that …

【修改】Certain biological changes associated with depression may lead to dementia.

2.3 语言含糊,缺乏准确性和规范性

例 3:

Mice in the control group and the model group had almost the same incidence of hypertension.

【分析】医学专业英语表达要求准确,学术报告中要避免使用表意含糊的词组,比如 almost the same,在表述科研结果时要么是相同的(the same)、完全相同的(identical),要么是相当的(equivalent)、相似的(similar)、可比的(comparable)。

【修改】Mice in the control group and the model group had an equivalent incidence of hypertension.

第三节　练习巩固

1. 找一篇专业领域的学术报告,标示出其中导言和结束语、内容与致谢语,以及提问与答复语用到的英文表达,并分析语言特征。

2. 修改以下学术报告中的句子。

（1）The CD57 expression on CD8＋ cells in certain viral infections，such as CMV and HIV，has been demonstrated.

（2）Excessive *in vitro* LPS-induced production of IL-i in chronic liver diseases and their correlation with hepatic fibrosis has been reported.

（3）The inhibitory effects of EGB and EGS(2.0 g · L^{-1}) on the generation of AGEs were almost the same as that of aminoguanidine at the same concentration.

（4）I think，this human 4-hr patch test could be a valid alternative to the rabbit test for the assessment of skin irritation.

参考文献

[1] 龚长华.实用医学英语写作教程[M].上海:世界图书出版公司,2014.

[2] 胡庚升.国际会议交流[M].北京:外语教学与研究出版社,2013.

[3] 黄萍.中国专门用途英语研究的发展与实践[M].北京:科学出版社,2020.

[4] 李传英,潘承礼.医学英语写作与翻译[M].武汉:武汉大学出版社,2014.

[5] 庞炜,刘维静.医学英语写作[M].南京:南京大学出版社,2013.

[6] 吴江梅,赵霞.医学英语论文写作[M].北京:中国人民大学出版社,2016.

[7] 伍斌,胡志清.汉语对中国英语学习者英语学术写作中外壳名词使用的影响研究[J].外语教育,
2018,04:72-82.

[8] 姚欣,龚修林.医学英语术语学教程[M].南京:南京大学出版社,2010.

[9] 殷红梅,张红芹.英文医学学术论文写作[M].南京:南京大学出版社,2021.

[10] 詹思延,王聪霞,孙凤.系统综述与 Meta 分析[M].北京:人民卫生出版社,2019.

[11] 张德禄,刘汝山.语篇连贯与衔接理论的发展及应用[M].第 2 版.上海:上海外语教育出版
社,2018.

[12] 张毓.学术文本概指名词的特征性型式与局部功能[M].上海:上海交通大学出版社,2020.

[13] AGGARWAL R, CHARLES-SCHOEMAN C, SCHESSL J, et al. Trial of intravenous immune
globulin in dermatomyositis[J]. N Engl J Med, 2022, 387(14): 1264 - 1278.

[14] ALEXANDER J H, et al. Apixaban with antiplatelet therapy after acute coronary syndrome[J].
N Engl J Med, 2011, 365(8):699 - 708.

[15] BAIER C, et al. Incidence and risk factors of surgical site infection after total knee arthroplasty:
Results of a retrospective cohort study[J]. American Journal of Infection Control, 2019, 47:
1270 - 1272.

[16] BATES D W, LEVINE D M, SALMASIAN H, et al. The safety of inpatient health care[J]. N
Engl J Med, 2023, 388(2): 142 - 153.

[17] BI M L, LI D Y, et al. Male axillary accessory breast cancer: A case report[J]. Medicine
(Baltimore), 2020, 99(11):e19506.

[18] BIRHAN A T. Effects of teaching lexical bundles on EFL students' abstract genre academic
writing skills improvement: Corpus-based research design[J]. International Journal of Language
Education, 2021, 01: 585 - 597.

[19] BJORNSTAD P, et al. Long-term complications in youth-onset type 2 diabetes[J]. Engl J Med,
2021, 385: 416 - 26.

[20] BOGOCH I I, et al. Assessment of the potential for international dissemination of Ebola virus
via commercial air travel during the 2014 west African outbreak[J]. Lancet, 2015, 385(9962):
29 - 35.

[21] BRETTHAUER M, LØBERG M, WIESZCZY P, et al. Effect of colonoscopy screening on risks of colorectal cancer and related death[J]. N Engl J Med, 2022, 387(17):1547 - 1556.

[22] BYRNE D W. Publishing your medical research paper[M]. 2nd ed. Philadelphia: Wolters Kluwer Health, 2017.

[23] CHOJNOWSKA S, et al. Human saliva as a diagnostic material[J]. Advances in Medical Sciences, 2018, 63: 185 - 191.

[24] CHOW Y K, et al. Limbic brain structures and burnout-A systematic review[J]. Advances in Medical Sciences, 2018, 63(1):192 - 198.

[25] DABELEA D, STAFFORD J M, MAYER-DAVIS E J, et al. Association of type 1 diabetes vs type 2 diabetes diagnosed during childhood and adolescence with complications during teenage years and young adulthood[J]. JAMA, 2017, 317(8): 825 - 835.

[26] DU F J, YANG M W, FANG J ZH, et al. Primary hepatic malignant melanoma: A case report [J]. Int J Clin Exp Pathol, 2015, 8(2): 2199 - 2201.

[27] DURDELLA H, EVERETT S, ROSE J A. Acute phlegmonous gastritis: A case report[J]. JACEP Open, 2022, 3: e12640.

[28] FITRIANASARI N V. Lexical bundles in academic writing by undergraduate and graduate students of English language education program[J]. Loquen: English Studies Journal, 2018, 2: 1 - 14.

[29] FRANCOIS B, et al. Prevention of early ventilator-associated pneumonia after cardiac arrest[J]. N Engl J Med, 2019, 381(19):1831 - 1842.

[30] FREUND Y, COHEN-AUBART F, BLOOM B. Acute pulmonary embolism: A review[J]. JAMA, 2022, 328(13): 1336 - 1345.

[31] GILLETT A, et al. Successful academic writing[M]. Harlow, UK: Pearson Longman, 2009.

[32] GLENDINNING E H, HOWARD R. Professional English in use: Medicine[M]. Beijing:Posts and Telecom Press, 2012.

[33] GOODWIN G M, et al. Single-dose psilocybin for a treatment-resistant episode of major depression[J]. N Engl J Med, 2022, 387:1637 - 1648.

[34] GOYAL S, et al. Bacterial contamination of medical providers' white coats and surgical scrubs: A systematic review[J]. Am J Infect Control, 2019, 47(8):994 - 1001.

[35] HAJEK P, et al. A randomized trial of E-cigarettes versus Nicotine-replacement therapy[J]. N Engl J Med, 2019, 380(7):629 - 637.

[36] HIDAKA B H. Depression as a disease of modernity: Explanations for increasing prevalence[J]. Journal of Affective Disorders, 2012, 3:205 - 214.

[37] HOOD R B, MILLER W C, SHOBEN A, et al. Maternal hepatitis C virus infection and adverse newborn outcomes in the US[J]. Matern Child Health J, 2023, 27(8):1343 - 1351.

[38] HU G SH. International confercommunication[M]. Beijing: Foreign Language Teaching and Research Press, 2013: 127.

[39] JACOBS M, RODGER A, BELL D J, et al. Late Ebola virus relapse causing meningoencephalitis: a case report[J]. Lancet, 2016, 388(10043):498 - 503.

[40] JIA J, ZHAO T, LIU Z, et al. Association between healthy lifestyle and memory decline in

older adults: 10 year, population based, prospective cohort study[J]. BMJ, 2023, 380:e072691.

[41] LIU C, CHEN R J, et al. Ambient particulate air pollution and daily mortality in 652 Cities[J]. N Engl J Med, 2019, 381(8): 705-715.

[42] LIU N, LI SH T, JIA J M. Advanced breast cancer with cachexia: A case report[J]. Medicine, 2021, 100(4): e24397.

[43] MEDRANO-ENGAY B, et al. Iron homeostasis and inflammatory biomarker analysis in patients with type 1 Gaucher disease[J]. Blood Cells, Molecules and Diseases, 2014, 53: 171-175.

[44] MILLER G D, et al. Hematological changes following an Ironman triathlon: An antidoping perspective[J]. Drug Test Anal, 2019, 11(11-12):1747-1754.

[45] MIRO-CZUK-CHODAKOWSKA I, WITKOWSKA A M, et al. Endogenous non-enzymatic antioxidants in the human body[J]. Advances in Medical Sciences, 2018, 63(1):68-78.

[46] MOHAMMED S H, et al. Neighbourhood socioeconomic status and overweight/obesity: a systematic review and meta-analysis of epidemiological studies[J]. BMJ Open, 2019, 9 (11): e028238.

[47] MONTECUCCO C, et al. Low-dose oral prednisone improves clinical and ultrasonographic remission rates in early rheumatoid arthritis: Results of a 12-month open-label randomised study [J]. Arthritis Research & Therapy, 2012,14(3): R112.

[48] NADERI M, COHAN N, et al. A retrospective study on clinical manifestations of neonates with FXIII-A deficiency[J]. Blood Cells, Molecules and Diseases, 2019, 77: 78-81.

[49] NIÑO J L G, WU H, LACOURSE K D, et al. Effect of the intratumoral microbiota on spatial and cellular heterogeneity in cancer[J]. Nature, 2022, 611(7937):810-817.

[50] NOORDIN N. The effects of electronic feedback on medical university students' writing performance[J]. International Journal of Higher Education, 2021, 4: 124-134.

[51] NUNDY S, et al. How to practice academic medicine and publish from developing countries? A practical guide[M]. Berlin: Springer, 2022.

[52] O'FLYNN J. Lexical bundles in the academic writing of the arts and humanities: from corpus to CALL[J]. De Gauyter Mouton, 2022, 13: 81-108.

[53] OKTAY K, HARVEY B E, PARTRIDGE A H, et al. Fertility preservation in patients with cancer: ASCO clinical practice guideline update[J]. J Clin Oncol, 2018, 36(19): 1994-2001.

[54] PATIBANDLA S A, PRABHAKAR B S. Autoimmunity to the thyroid stimulating hormone receptor[J]. Advances in Neuroimmunology, 1996, 6(4): 347-57.

[55] PERERA D, CLAYTON T, O'KANE P D, et al. Percutaneous revascularization for ischemic left ventricular dysfunction[J]. N Engl J Med, 2022, 387(15): 1351-1360.

[56] POOL, R. A corpus-aided approach for the teaching and the learning of rhetoric in an undergraduate course for L2 writers[J]. Journal of English for Academic Purposes, 2016, 21: 99-109.

[57] QUAIL Z, CARTER M M, WEI A, LI X. Management of cognitive decline in Alzheimer's disease using a non-pharmacological intervention program: A case report[J]. Medicine, 2020, 99: 21(e20128).

[58] SHARMA A, et al. Case 25 – 2020: A 47-year-old woman with a lung mass[J]. N Engl J Med, 2020, 383: 665 – 674.

[59] STIELL I G, NICHOL G, et al. Early versus later rhythm analysis in patients with out-of-hospital cardiac arrest [J]. N Engl J Med, 2011, 365(9):787 – 97.

[60] SUN D, LIU Y L. The use of English preposition with in essays written by Chinese EFL learners[J]. Lecture Notes in Arts and Humanities (ICCLAH2021), 2021, 4: 107 – 110.

[61] SZUHANY K L, SIMON N M. Anxiety Disorders: A Review[J]. JAMA, 2022, 328(24): 2431 – 2445.

[62] TANAKA H, HAYASHI A, MORIMOTO T, et al. A case of lung adenocarcinoma harboring EGFR mutation and EML4-ALK fusion gene[J]. BMC Cancer, 2012,12: 558.

[63] THAKKAR D, KATE A S. Update on metabolism of Abemaciclib: In Silico, in vitro and in vivo metabolite identification and characterization using High Resolution Mass spectrometry[J]. Drug Test Anal, 2020, 12(3): 331 – 342.

[64] TOELLE B G, et al. Respiratory symptoms and illness in older Australians: the Burden of Obstructive Lung Disease (BOLD) study[J]. The Medical Journal of Australia, 2013, 198(3): 144 – 148.

[65] VILLANUEVA C, et al. Transfusion Strategies for Acute Upper Gastrointestinal Bleeding[J]. N Engl J Med, 2013, 368:11 – 21.

[66] WALKER M D, SHANE E. Hypercalcemia: A review[J]. JAMA, 2022, 328(16):1624 – 1636.

[67] WU B, YU ZH W, et al. Evaluation of small dense low-density lipoprotein concentration for predicting the risk of acute coronary syndrome in Chinese population[J]. Journal of Clinical Laboratory Analysis, 2020, 34(3): e23085.

[68] WU Y, GUI S Y, et al. Exposure to outdoor light and risk of breast cancer: A systematic review and meta-analysis of observational studies[J]. Environmental Pollution, 2021, 269:114 – 116.

[69] XU X F, XING H, et al. Risk factors, patterns, and outcomes of late recurrence after liver resection for hepatocellualr carcinoma: A multicenter study from China[J]. JAMA Surg, 2019, 154(3):209 – 217.

[70] ZANNAD F, et al. Eplerenone in patients with systolic heart failure and Mmild symptoms[J]. N Engl J Med, 2011, 364(1): 11 – 21.